Prai

"I'm a baseball fan, but even more important, I'm a great believer in the fact that you can tell a lot about character when the going gets tough. [Dave Dravecky] showed us real courage—so did [his] wife."

—President George Bush

"The remarkable faith and courage [Dave Dravecky] has shown is an inspiration to us all. Dave has many friends and fans around the country, and Nancy and I are proud to be among them."

—Ronald Reagan

"Baseball people say that anybody can field a good hop. The test is how a player handles a bad hop. Life gave Dave Dravecky a bad hop. In COMEBACK Dave tells us how he handled it. His story is must reading."

—Joe Garagiola
Sports Analyst and Commentator

"[Dave Dravecky's] has to be one of the great stories in baseball or anywhere, because it is truly an inspiration—what [he] has done . . . I still marvel at how he accepted the frustration, the pain, the disappointment, and put it all in the right perspective."

—Vin Scully
NBC *Sports* Commentator

DAVE DRAVECKY
COMEBACK

WITH TIM STAFFORD

HarperPaperbacks
A Division of HarperCollinsPublishers

To Janice

*To be blessed with the most precious
of all gems is truly a gift from God.
You are the wind beneath my wings.*

If you purchased this book without a cover, you should
be aware that this book is stolen property. It was reported as "unsold and destroyed" to the publisher and
neither the author nor the publisher has received any
payment for this "stripped book."

HarperPaperbacks   *A Division of* HarperCollins*Publishers*
10 East 53rd Street, New York, N.Y. 10022

Copyright © 1990 by Dave Dravecky
All rights reserved. No part of this book may be used
or reproduced in any manner whatsoever without written permission of the publisher, except in the case of
brief quotations embodied in critical articles and re-
views. For information address Zondervan Publishing
House, 1415 Lake Drive, S.E., Grand Rapids, Michigan
49508.

Credits appear following page 269.

A hardcover edition of this book was co-published in
1990 by Zondervan Publishing House and Harper &
Row Publishers, San Francisco.

First HarperPaperbacks printing: July 1991

Printed in the United States of America

HarperPaperbacks and colophon are trademarks of
HarperCollins*Publishers*

10 9 8 7 6 5 4 3 2 1

Contents

COMEBACK

Chronology of Events

June, 1978. Dave Dravecky graduates from Youngstown State University and is drafted by the Pittsburgh Pirates in the twenty-first round.

October 7, 1978. Dravecky marries Janice Roh.

April, 1979. Dravecky is sent by the Pittsburgh Pirates to the Double-A Buffalo Bisons, where he plays for the next two seasons.

December, 1979. Dave and Janice leave Barranquilla, Colombia, after two months of winter ball.

October, 1980. Dravecky returns to Barranquilla, Colombia, for another season of winter ball.

COMEBACK

April, 1981. Traded to the San Diego Padres' organization, Dravecky is sent to Amarillo, Texas, for his third year in Double-A baseball.

June 6, 1982. Tiffany Dravecky is born in Honolulu, Hawaii, where Dave Dravecky is pitching for San Diego's Triple-A tea. Two days later the San Diego Padres call up Dravecky to the major leagues.

July 6, 1983. Dravecky is chosen to represent the National League in the All-Star game, and pitches two scoreless innings.

October, 1984. Dravecky makes five relief appearances for the San Diego Padres in the National League championships and the World Series, pitching ten and two-thirds scoreless innings.

January 8, 1985. Jonathan Dravecky is born in San Diego California.

July 4, 1987. Dravecky is traded to the San Francisco Giants along with Kevin Mitchell and Craig Lefferts.

October 7, 1987. Dravecky pitches in the National League championship series against the St. Louis Cardinals, and wins 5-0.

January 26, 1988. Tests indicate that a lump on Dravecky's left arm is probably benign.

April 4, 1988. Dravecky pitches opening day against the Los Angeles Dodgers, winning 5-1.

Chronology of Events

June 11, 1988. Arthroscopic surgery on Dravecky's left shoulder puts him on the disabled list for the rest of the 1988 season.

September 19, 1988. Dr. George Muschler of the Cleveland Clinic indicates that Dravecky's lump may be cancerous, and a biopsy is needed.

October 7, 1988. Surgery removes one-half of the deltoid muscle in Dravecky's pitching arm. To kill all cancerous cells, part of the humerus bone is frozen.

January 9, 1989. Doctors at the Cleveland Clinic give the okay for throwing a football, and plan a rehabilitation schedule that could bring Dravecky back to pitch by midsummer.

May, 1989. Because Dravecky's shoulder is hurting and he has "hit the wall," he is put on total rest for one month.

July 8, 1989. In St. Louis, Dravecky pitches his first simulated game.

July 23, 1989. Dravecky pitches for the Class-A San Jose Giants in Stockton, California, before 4,200 fans. He pitches a complete game and wins 2-0.

July 28, 1989. Pitching again for San Jose, Dravecky wins a complete game in Reno, 7-3.

COMEBACK

August 4, 1989. Moving to Triple-A Phoenix, Dravecky leads the Firebirds over Tucson, 3-2, in a complete-game seven-hitter.

August 10, 1989. Dravecky pitches his first major league game in more than a year going for eight innings against the Cincinnati Reds, and winning 4-3.

August 15, 1989. While pitching in Montreal, Dravecky's humerus bone snaps.

October 9, 1989. While celebrating victory in the National League championship series, Dravecky's arm is broken again.

October 17, 1989. An earthquake stops the World Series.

October 27, 1989. Doctors at the Cleveland Clinic tell Dravecky that cancer has probably recurred in his arm.

November 13, 1989. Dravecky announces his retirement from baseball.

Foreword

By the rude bridge that arched the flood,
Their flag to April's breeze unfurled,
Here once the embattled farmers stood,
And fired the shot heard round the world.

Ralph Waldo Emerson's immortal words gave
birth to the hymn our forebears sang on July 4,
1837, at the completion of the battle monument in
Concord. I have stood at the Old Concord Bridge
and mentally replayed that epochal moment. All
who have done so can almost hear the initial blast
of gunpowder and see the burst of fire explode
from the farmer's musket. Little did the unnamed
hero realize the far-reaching impact his shot would
make when he took aim and squeezed the trigger.
Nothing would ever be the same. What was to him
merely his duty as a patriot has become the point
on which our country's history pivots. His was in-
deed "the shot heard round the world."

The book you are about to read is the true ac-
count of another history-making event . . . not
brought about by guns and soldiers, but quietly
modeled in the life of a man whose name is now
well-known because of his courageous faith. Dave
Dravecky's story is not just another athlete's story,

because Dave is not just another athlete. His major struggles have not been limited to locker rooms and pitcher's mounds. And though he has known the thrill of playing a vital role on a championship major league baseball team, his greatest victories have not been won in public ballparks. His most significant conquests have come deep within his own life as he refused to surrender to the same enemies that plague us all: fear and disappointment, pain and death.

A curious swelling no larger than a quarter on Dave's pitching arm was diagnosed as a malignant tumor. Yet his determination mixed with optimism following surgery and therapy got him back into the game. The whole sports world watched in amazement as the all-star hurler returned to the mound, confident and sure as ever. Many called it a miracle as he was reunited with his team, the San Francisco Giants. In early August of '89, amid repeated, thunderous applause, he earned a decisive win against the Cincinnati Reds. As he lifted his cap for a final bow following that incredible achievement, he received his twelfth standing ovation of the day. Everybody who was anybody in the world of news had his name on their lips. Dave Dravecky was suddenly a synonym for *comeback.*

His next game was in Montreal. Excitement was at an all-time high. Throwing with a strange tingling sensation in his arm, Dave pitched well enough through five innings to be ahead 3—0, a nice cushion to enjoy. In the bottom of the sixth, he faced a tough hitter at the plate, Tim Raines. Dave took his set, stared at first base to restrain a runner, pivoted, and kicking high, he pushed off the rubber and let fly. He didn't realize it would be the last pitch of his life. A dull, sickening crack could be heard across the unusually quiet stadium. The humerus bone in his pitching arm literally snapped as he delivered with full force. In Dave's own words, "My arm felt like I'd been hit with a meat axe." He grabbed his arm to keep it from flying toward home plate as he screamed, tumbling headfirst to the ground.

It was enough to devastate the strongest of the strong. Not Dave Dravecky. Remarkable though it may seem today, his thoughts were not full of bitterness or self-pity. Rather, he found himself overflowing with gratitude, confident that God was writing another chapter in his life. Something more, something amazing was about to be revealed. At the time he had no idea what it was. Little did he realize, as he writhed in pain upon the ground, that he had delivered "the pitch heard round the world."

Now he does. And that's why *Comeback* has been written.

Chuck Swindoll
Pastor

Acknowledgments

Writing a book has been a completely new experience for me, one I could never have managed without others' help. My literary agents, Sealy Yates and Rick Christian, came into my life as a godsend, relieving pressure on me over the decision about publishers. Sealy, in particular, has become a close friend—someone I look to for advice, someone whose wisdom I trust. The staff of Zondervan Publishing House, particularly John Sloan, my editor, and Scott Bolinder, my publisher, have been tremendously helpful. I am especially grateful for the superb writing assistance of Tim Stafford, who helped me bring my experiences to life in the following pages. I believe God put together a team of friends to make this book possible.

In addition to thanking those who helped me put this book together, I'd like to acknowledge those who helped me in the comeback this book is all about. I particularly want to thank my teammates on the San Francisco Giants, whose support and encouragement I could count on every day. Manager Roger Craig and his coaching staff, trainers Mark Letendre and Greg Lynn, and many others in the Giants organization stood behind me, rooting for me and helping me. The Giants' front office, led by Bob Lurie and Al Rosen, offered me complete freedom to work at my own pace, and an unending willingness to help in any way they could. Pat and Joan Gallagher were particularly involved in introducing me to Alex Vlahos, adding a caring dimension to the business of baseball. Special thanks also to the Giants' chapel coordinator, Pat Richie, and his wife Nico for their spiritual encouragement.

I would also like to thank the San Diego Padres, including its staff and fans, for five and a half truly memorable, unforgettable years. Even though I eventually became a pitcher for the San Francisco Giants, I left a big chunk of my heart in San Diego.

So many people have played a part in my comeback that I could never mention all those I'd like to. But I want to mention those who have meant the most to me. My mom and dad, and my brothers, Rick, Frankie, Joe, and George, have loved me through thick and thin. Any time I needed help, day or night, I knew they would be there. Special thanks also to Janice's brother Randy Roh and his wife Kim for their prayers and support during this time.

Dr. Mark Roh, Janice's cousin, counseled Janice and me as we found our way through many confusing and difficult medical questions. We knew he would see that we were taken care of in the best possible way.

Dr. George Muschler, my doctor at the Cleveland Clinic, cared for me and Janice as though we were members of his own family. Dr. Murray Brennan and his staff have also provided critical care for me, and I know I can look to them with confidence in the days ahead. Other doctors and medical personnel also played crucial roles, particularly Dr. John Bergfeld and his staff, Dr. Gordon Campbell and his staff, and my physical therapists Larry Brown and Ken Johnson.

Long before my adventure with cancer began, Bryon Ballard gave me the greatest gift one man can give another: he introduced me to Jesus, my Lord and my God. Myles Gentzkow and Larry Dean have been my spiritual mentors, helping me grow and mature. Many, many others have given themselves to me by caring, by taking the time to call, by sharing words of encouragement, by praying. The members of Tabernacle Evangelical Presbyterian Church particularly supported Janice and me.

I have been blessed with deep friendships, and I believe this book witnesses to their significance in my life. Here I would like merely to mention my deep love for three couples that mean the world to me: Atlee and Jenny Hammaker, Scott and Kathy Garrelts, and Bob and Teri Knepper.

All these people, and many more, have contributed to my life. I owe them more than I can say. To Jesus Christ be the glory.

Prologue

BY looks, baseball is a nineteenth-century antique, what with its old-timey uniforms, complete with tiny caps. By feel, it has the slowness and gravity we imagine in our nation's past. The game is over when it is over, whether it be two hours after the beginning or four. An inning can last five minutes or fifty.

So why does baseball survive? By look and feel it belongs with croquet, played occasionally for memory's sake on picnics.

Baseball survives, and thrives, because it is a game in which we see ourselves. The players are not huge brutes, dressed like gladiators. They look to be of a normal size and strength. Their skill is not obvious, either. Hitting a baseball may be the most difficult athletic feat of all, but it does not look hard. Very rarely in baseball does somebody make a play that appears impossible for mortals. (It happens every day in basketball.)

In the imagination, then, baseball lets us live our dreams. That is what gives the story in this book its special flavor. It is the story of a comeback, a comeback in baseball, a sport which has become a metaphor for the American dream.

1

COMEBACK

Here is Dave Dravecky, standing on the pitcher's mound, looking high into the stands mounting up to the sky filled with cheering, shouting, whistling, stomping ecstasy. What has he done to deserve this adoration? He has not yet thrown a pitch. The game has not even yet begun, and though this is mid-August, Dave Dravecky has not yet thrown in the major leagues this year.

What has he done to deserve such a welcome?

He has come back. He has heard the experts say he can never do it. Yet in spite of their doubts, he has come back.

The fans cheer for Dave Dravecky because they too face difficulty, and by all odds will not overcome it. Yet they cannot help hoping, and believing. What Dave Dravecky has done, before he even throws a pitch, is to validate their hope. Yes, it is possible. Yes, you can come back.

—Tim Stafford

Between the Lines

TO fully understand baseball, you must pay attention to little things. Everyone knows it when Will Clark cranks a home run into the stands. That's big and noisy and obvious. Yet often a game is decided because of a much quieter event: a two-out walk, for example, that barely stirs a ripple in the ranks of sprawling, sunbaked spectators. They paid their money to see home runs; they barely notice walks.

But players and coaches notice. They know too well how an insignificant walk can be the first tiny tear in the fabric of a close game, like a rip in the seam of a tightly stuffed pillow. Open the seam and, before you know it, stuffing is all over the place.

A two-out walk, or a pop fly that drops into a tiny open triangle of green that the second baseman, first baseman, and right fielder converge on just a second too late, or a tame ground ball that somehow maddeningly hops between the diving second baseman and the diving shortstop—each of these small events is like an open invitation: Chaos, come on in! Baseball players sit up and take note of little things. Often a close game is de-

3

cided by one of those sneaky little insignificant happenings that set off a chain reaction.

I am what is called a finesse pitcher. I do not have overpowering stuff. My fastball rarely reaches ninety miles per hour, and my slider doesn't break a foot. I get outs by surprising batters, by keeping them off balance, and by putting the ball within an inch or two of where I intend it. I use small distances, which make small differences in batters' swings, which result in weak ground balls or pop flies. Finesse pitchers pay attention to little things. In fact, all real pitchers—as opposed to mere throwers—do.

Cancer came into my life as a small thing. I first noticed the lump in the fall of 1987.

When, exactly, I do not even know. Running my hand along my left arm, I found a firm, round shape under the skin on the upper arm, about the size of a quarter. It didn't hurt. It didn't show. And I paid it little attention. That lump, which was to create so much turmoil in my life, made almost no impression on me at all.

It was sometime in September. The regular season was almost over, and we had clinched the division title. The games went on, of course—we still had to play every day—but our thoughts were elsewhere. Roger Craig, the folksy, crafty manager of my team, the San Francisco Giants, was preparing the pitching rotation to face the St. Louis Cardinals in the playoffs. It was a time of intense but quiet anticipation, the pause before the carnival. We were making ready for what every baseball player works for, and most never experience: postseason play. That's when baseball takes off its everyday work clothes and puts on a party outfit. The stands are draped in red-white-and-blue bunting, the "Star Spangled Banner" is sung by star musicians rather than ground out on an organ, and the regular print reporters rub shoulders with media stars like Vin Scully and Joe Garagiola. The colors are brighter in the postseason. The prices double yet fans feel blessed if they get a ticket.

So I had other things on my mind than a little, painless lump. As a matter of fact, my arm felt the best it had in years. During many of my six seasons with the San Diego Padres my elbow had been sore. Since coming to the Giants on July 4, along with Kevin Mitchell and Craig Lefferts, my arm had recovered. I was nearly pain-free. I felt on top of my game.

It was a curious little lump, unlike anything I had experienced before. In the training room one day, deep in the concrete bowels of Candlestick Park, I happened to think of it. It was quiet in the clubhouse, as it usually is. As I was going out the door, I approached our trainer, Mark Letendre.

"Hey, Mark, take a look at this little lump. It doesn't hurt, but I thought I should draw it to your attention."

Mark ran his fingers over my arm, kneading the flesh. "Don't worry about it," he said. And I didn't.

There are many aspects of professional baseball I could happily live without. I hate the travel. To the bottom of my being I despise being separated from my family. For six months of the year you're on the road exactly fifty percent of the time, and even when you're home most of the games are at night. I generally leave for the ballpark at two in the afternoon, and arrive home after midnight. I get used to that schedule, but my kids don't. While school is on they're coming home about the time that I leave for work.

Then I take off with the team for two weeks of travel. When I get home from a long road trip, my kids often won't speak to me. Tiffany is a beautiful little seven-year-old, and Jonathan, at four, looks like my carbon copy. I'll come in the door and hold out my arms for a big hug, and for the first half hour they'll act like I'm a repairman. It's like they're saying, "You left me here with my love, and you didn't come back for two weeks, and now you expect me to give you a hug and a kiss. Well, forget it."

They get over it, eventually, and decide to forgive me. But not before they've made their point.

My wife Janice, on the other hand, understands what I'm doing, and why. She's always been very supportive. Nevertheless, she isn't completely delighted with life as a single parent when I'm gone. She's proud of my baseball career, but she could do happily without the lifestyle.

Yes, baseball offers fame and fortune. I'm thankful for it—I'm certainly glad to be able to provide well for my family while playing a game I love. But there's a down side to it. Adulation and wealth help create an unreal atmosphere. Some players begin to think that baseball—and life—owes them everything. Athletes are no better than the rest of mankind, and the pressures and temptations athletes live with may be harder. A major league clubhouse is a long way from heaven. I'd give it up without a second thought. Even the fame and money—I'd give them up, and I really don't think I'd regret it.

What I could not so easily give up is the game. That's what I love. I love to walk between the lines—across those narrow stripes of chalk that begin at the corners of home plate and extend out across green grass to the fences. Within those lines is the game I love to play. I have a passion for it.

Baseball is a team sport, but I think the nature of that teamwork is often misunderstood. Each play is one on one: man against man, or man against ball. It's what you do individually that contributes to the team. I love that: the individual challenges.

When I'm really locked in, I hardly know who is hitting. I know how I want to pitch to the guy, I've thought about his weaknesses all season, but when he walks to the plate that's faded into the background. The seven men behind me hardly exist either. Of course I'm counting on them, but I'm not thinking about them. My focus is in a tunnel between me and my catcher. All I'm seeing is him and the target he puts down. That's my zone. That's where I compete. I'm not thinking about blowing away any particular batter, besting him, showing him up. I'm really hardly aware of who he is. My challenge is to put the ball where I want to put it, into that tiny pocket of the catcher's glove.

I started the second game of the '87 National League playoffs in St. Louis. It was a day game, clean and crisp as October can be. In the long, autumn shadows the air was chilly, and fans wore winter coats. But on the field, where we stretched and shagged flies and hit batting practice before the game, the bright sunlight felt wonderful.

The Cardinals' stadium, a sparkling clean, modern oval, was buzzing with the kind of excitement you feel only in the postseason. Most of the year, a baseball game is significant only because it puts up a win or a loss for the team. Nobody remembers the details. In postseason, every pitch, every swing, every foul ball seems to be meant for the history books.

I love to pitch in the Cardinals' ballpark. It's a wonderful stadium, the fans are terrific, and the team management treats players like royalty. Also, I love to pitch under pressure. I've never been a guy who pitches his best while warming up—what we call a bull pen pitcher. You ask my catcher what kind of stuff I have warming up, he's likely to tell you he hopes I last through the first inning. That doesn't bother me at all. So long as I've got my rhythm and balance, I don't care if I'm bouncing fifty-five-foot fastballs in the bull pen. I know when I walk between the lines it will be different. I need the pressure, and I love it. The postseason is pure pressure.

I came down the runway into the open air of the playing field feeling all fired up. We had lost the first game to St. Louis, by a score of 5 to 3. It is commonly believed in baseball that to lose the first two games of a seven-game series is suicide. To have any hope of going on to the World Series, we had to win the second game. I would be opposing

John Tudor, one of the outstanding pitchers in baseball.

Besides everything else, it was my wedding anniversary. What a day.

I wasn't nervous. Excited, yes, but not really nervous. As soon as I got on the mound and threw my first pitch, I became totally absorbed by the game. My vision closed down. I saw my catcher, Bob Melvin. I saw his glove. I didn't see much else.

Baseball can seem to move slowly, and then with the speed of an accident, the game changes character. In the top of the second inning, Candy Maldonado, our right fielder, led off with a crisp single. He was followed by Will Clark, who with a long, smooth, effortless ellipse of his bat locked on a pitch and sent it high in the air to right field. Jose Oquendo backed up to the fence, as though he had a bead on it, and Candy went back to first base to tag up. But the ball fell into the stands for a home run. Suddenly, with hardly any warning, we were ahead 2–0. Busch Stadium fell absolutely quiet.

I kept it quiet. The *San Francisco Chronicle* wrote of my pitching that day, "It was so easy it seemed effortless. It was so effortless it seemed boring." Perhaps so, but not to me. I was pitching the game of my life. Every time the 55,331 fans stirred to life, I quieted them. There on the mound, throwing my pitches, I was able to completely control the mood and the tempo of the game. It was an incredible feeling of power.

Here's how to tell whether I'm pitching at my best: Watch how many bats I break. When my slider is perfectly placed, it comes at a right-handed batter as though it were off the outside corner of the plate. Then at the last second, when he's decided not to swing, the pitch breaks down and in, onto the outside corner. That's called a backdoor slider.

It sets up my fastball inside. The batter who's seen that slider on the outside corner is leaning out over the plate. A fastball on the inside corner catches him leaning too far. He swings, but he's hitting on the thin part of the bat, and it shatters.

That day I broke five bats.

In the fourth inning, our left fielder Jeffrey Leonard came to the plate. The Cardinal fans had taken a dislike to Jeffrey, possibly because he had been hitting a home run a day, and rounding the bases with all the quickness of a four-wheel-drive vehicle in deep mud. The fans taunted Jeffrey with a high, mocking call: Jeff-REE! Jeff-REE!

Leonard is a strong, proud, tough-looking dude. He fouled off a few pitches and then went deep to straightaway center field. The ball seemed to take a very long time to settle over the fence, and Leonard took even longer to circle the bases. It was 3–0. Busch Stadium was silent, as quiet as though everyone had just up and left.

As far as I was concerned, they might have. I was locked in. Fifty thousand fans did not exist to me. Even the batters barely existed. Only my catcher was there. We were thinking in sync, two, three pitches ahead. He knew what I wanted to throw. I knew that he knew. Some of the time we didn't even use signs. Pitches were called by lip service. If the count was 0 and 2, he knew my next pitch would be a fastball inside. Then I'd come back with the backdoor slider. When the batter wasn't looking I mouthed the words to Bob: "Backdoor." Bang! It was there, creasing the imaginary black line on the outside of the plate. Next batter.

In the top of the fifth inning, we almost broke it open. I even got a hit. But we blew a squeeze play and didn't score. The fans began to buzz. The momentum seemed to shift. The Cardinals were coming to life.

I went out to the mound thinking, *Keep on cheering. Make a little more noise. Because the silence will be that much greater when we're done with this inning.*

I was stoked. Not that you would know it by looking at me. My confidence doesn't come through in my expressions. If anything, I want to keep the fire out of my eyes, so my opponents don't see what I'm feeling.

But I was confident to my bones. It gave me a feeling I can't describe in words, to go out there with the crowd stirring and beginning to chant, and to put them back to sleep.

We scored twice more in the eighth inning, thanks to a very rare error by Ozzie Smith. Ozzie glided toward third base for a ground ball, made an effortless dip to the carpet—and came up empty. The ball hopped between his legs, and, running full speed, two men scored. With a five-run lead I coasted home with my first postseason win. I'd given up two hits and no runs, putting myself in the record books. In the 1984 playoffs and World Series I'd pitched five times in relief and not given up a run. Now I'd run my postseason record to nineteen and two-thirds scoreless innings.

COMEBACK

*   *   *

After the game I was summoned to the interview room. Usually the press talk to you by your locker. At most, a small handful of reporters gather around you there. But for postseason play there are so many reporters present that they set up a special room with a microphone for a few key players.

I walked in late, while Roger Craig was talking in his John Wayne drawl. The room was jammed with reporters holding their tape recorders into the air, with TV cameramen vying for elbow room, with bright lights. I could barely get through the crush.

Apparently somebody had asked Roger a question about Christian ballplayers. There's a common rap on Christians, that they are too nice to be winners, that they just shrug their shoulders and praise the Lord when they lose, and so lack the intensity and determination to come through in tough games. I was shouldering my way to the front of the room when I heard Roger say, "They say Christians don't have any guts. Well, this guy's a Christian and he's not afraid of anything." That was his introduction. He handed the microphone over to me.

Right away a writer from one of the big papers followed up. "Roger just commented about what some people say, that Christian athletes don't have guts. How do you respond to that?"

You have to understand how rare an opportunity that is. Most of the time reporters are very careful not to ask you anything that might lead into the subject of religion. If you were to talk about how you get inspiration from your pet beagle, they would be interested in that, but when God comes into the picture reporters generally steer far away. They quickly go on to another subject, and you can be pretty sure any words about faith won't be quoted.

In some ways I can appreciate their motives. A person's faith in God is a very personal matter. But I'd really like to be able to tell people about who I am and what matters most to me, if they want to know. So I was delighted at that moment, with the eyes of America on me, on live TV, to be asked that question.

They were asking, essentially, whether Christians are wimps. The best way to answer that question, I thought, was to ask whether Jesus was a wimp. After all, Christians are followers of Jesus. If he was a wimp, Christians should be too.

I told them that if Jesus were in my shoes, called to compete as a professional athlete, he would be the best athlete on the field. He would play with more intensity and aggressiveness than any other athlete. But he would always be under control.

I didn't mean to suggest that I picture Jesus as a baseball player. Jesus had more important things to do than to play baseball. But in whatever Jesus did, whether preaching to crowds or caring for a single, insignificant individual, he did it uncompromisingly, intensely, and powerfully. As anybody who has read the Bible knows, Jesus was no wimp. So if I imagine Jesus doing the job I'm called to do, I can easily imagine him doing it in a way I would have to respect.

I said to the reporters, "Jesus Christ is my example. I play for him. When I play, I play to glorify God. I recognize the ability he's given me, and so I play with everything I have."

I loved getting the chance to tell them that.

I remember meeting my wife Janice after coming out of the clubhouse. She was in the long, crowded corridor where players' family members wait after the game.

I caught a glimpse of her through all the noisy, happy confusion of families greeting each other. She looked wonderful. Her face was glowing. I grabbed her and we kissed. When I told her about the postgame interview, she practically jumped up and down.

It was our ninth anniversary. I'd pitched a shut-out in the playoffs. I'd had a chance to give credit where credit is due—to God. Janice looked at me with stars in her eyes. She said, "I don't know how you're going to top this."

In Preparation

WHAT could top that? If I'd stopped to think seriously about what Janice had said, I suppose I might have thought of winning another playoff game, or of starting in the World Series.

That was not to be. We went home to Candlestick Park and won two out of the next three games. That meant we returned to St. Louis, needing only to win one of the last two. I started the first game; my best friend Atlee Hammaker was to pitch the second, if necessary. Atlee had done well in his first starting game, but the bull pen had blown his lead after he'd left. He'd had no decision.

I was quite relaxed before I pitched, as I usually am. I remember coming down the runway into the ballpark with Atlee. It was a concrete tunnel, dimly lit, underneath the stands. Atlee kept telling me, "You've got to win this one for us, Dave. You've got to win."

I told him, "Hey, it's no big deal, Atlee. If I don't win today, you'll win tomorrow."

It was a night game, cold and still. Overhead, above the lights, the sky was utterly black. Banks of lights held us all in a glow—players, umpires, coaches, fifty thousand fans—as though we were in a space station orbiting in perfect darkness.

My pitching that night was better than in my first playoff game. I didn't walk a man, and I struck out eight in six innings. The damage was all done by one of those little things.

In the second inning, Cardinal catcher Tony Pena led off with a weak line drive to right field, a routine catch for Candy Maldonado. But Candy hesitated, came in, made a feet-first slide—and missed the ball completely. It banged off his shoulder and rolled away, and by the time Chili Davis ran it down from his center field position, Pena had coasted into third.

Candy had lost the ball in the lights. It's one of those bizarre things that happens occasionally in baseball. At that point, in the second inning, it didn't seem like such a big deal. After all, we had been hitting Cardinal pitching like crazy.

I got Willie McGee to hit into a ground out, and Pena—who isn't terribly speedy—had to hold at third. Jose Oquendo came up. He hit a shallow fly ball down the right field line, which Candy raced for and caught. Pena was tagging up and heading for home. I was already there, backing up the throw.

Candy had to turn his body halfway around to throw. Maybe he tried a little too hard to make it good. The ball bounced off-line on the third-base side. Bob Melvin, our catcher, caught it and tried a whirling, diving tag, but he couldn't quite get there. Pena scored what turned out to be the only run of the game. It was also the only run ever scored off me in postseason play. One little run because of a fluke play. John Tudor pitched brilliantly against us. We lost 1–0.

The next night Atlee went out and got hit hard. For the second night in a row our team couldn't score a single run. And before we knew it we were on our way home to lick our wounds and watch the other guys play the World Series.

Janice and I, with our daughter Tiffany and son Jonathan, went home to San Diego. Losing to the Cardinals was tough, but it wasn't very long before the loss was swallowed up by very positive memories of the season. I had pitched the best games of my life in the most important games of my life. I'd given up just one run in two starting appearances, and that run, though it was scored as earned, obviously wasn't. As a team, we'd had a tremendous 1987 season. Just getting into the league championship series was a privilege.

Janice and I were ready to coast through that winter. We practically grew up together—we were high school sweethearts—and the passion for being together has really never been lacking, thank God. For us, the chance to catch up on each other after a long season was sheer joy.

Occasionally one of us would notice the lump on my arm and wonder about it, but it never occurred to us to worry. Even Janice, who is a planner and likes to nail down every detail about the future, wasn't thinking about that little lump.

We made some major decisions that winter, though, that turned out to affect the way we handled that lump. In particular, we decided to move back home.

COMEBACK

I'd said I'd never go back to Youngstown, Ohio, where both Janice and I grew up and went to college. When you're young, sometimes you want to get away and form your own identity. Through the minor leagues we'd lived all over America, and in some foreign countries, too. We'd settled in California, we were happy there, and we expected to stay.

But that Thanksgiving found us feeling as homesick as can be. Since we weren't with the San Diego Padres any more, we didn't have so many natural baseball connections. Our newly found friends among the Giants were far away. And maybe we realized that somewhere deep in our beings we weren't truly Californians. We'd been born and brought up in the Midwest. Nearly all our family members were still in Youngstown. Our children's grandparents and aunts and uncles were there. We knew that in Youngstown the weather would be crisp, perfect for building a fire and putting our feet up to the hearth. In San Diego, the Thanksgiving weather would be okay for the beach.

To be honest, Janice had been wanting to move home for some time. I had never been open to it. Every time she brought it up, I said I wanted to stay where we were.

But the day after Thanksgiving, when the kids had been put to bed and we were relaxing on the sofa in our family room, Janice looked up at me. "What are we doing here?" she asked.

I didn't know what she meant.

"What are we doing in San Diego? You work in San Francisco, our family's in Ohio, and we live in San Diego? It doesn't make sense. Let's move home."

She didn't really expect to get anywhere with that. She'd tried it before. This time, though, I thought for about ten seconds and said, "You're right."

Right there and then we decided. Within days we had a "For Sale" sign in front of our house. (We'd owned it six months, and lived in it for about two.) Over Christmas in Boardman, the suburb of Youngstown where I grew up and went to high school, where my parents still live and my brothers help run my dad's machine shop, we bought a beautiful lot. We hired an architect and told him to go to work. It was a decision that felt right. How right, we would discover later on.

During that off-season in San Diego I worked out at the Renaissance, a fitness center owned by the Nick Hoslag family. One day in January, out of the clear blue, I said to Nick, Sr., "Hey, Nick, come here and see the lump I've got on my arm."

There's something I don't completely understand here. So far as I can remember, I was never worried about that lump. Neither was Janice. Never once did we think that it might be serious. Yet my friends and family members remember me paying a lot of attention to it. I was always showing it to them, asking them to feel it. Maybe that shows I was subconsciously concerned. I certainly wasn't *consciously* concerned.

Nick came over and felt the lump on my arm, and he called his wife over and she felt it too. Then their son, Nick, Jr., came over. He said, "Hey, if I were you I wouldn't mess around with that. Why don't you have somebody check it?"

I told them that the Giants' trainer had looked at it. I said, "It doesn't hurt. It's no big deal." I appreciated their concern, but I didn't really want to make a big deal out of it.

But they said, "It's nothing to get a test done. Why don't you call the Giants and get permission? You can have the San Diego Padres' doctor do it."

A plastic surgeon was working out that day, and they asked him to come over and have a look. Obviously, he couldn't tell anything just from feeling the lump, but he agreed with them. He said, "If I were you, I'd get it checked."

It was hard to tell whether that lump had grown in the four months since I'd first noticed it. I thought it had, a little. But still I figured it was only a bad bruise from some bump I couldn't remember—that some scar tissue had calcified in there.

Reluctantly taking their advice, I got it checked by the Padres' orthopedic surgeons, Dr. Caldwell and Dr. Hirschman. On January 22, 1988, I went to the Scripps Clinic for a CAT scan, and four days later I went back for an MRI (Magnetic Resonance Image).

Getting it checked was not exactly "nothing." An MRI makes you feel like an experiment done in a science fiction movie. Because of its powerful magnet, the MRI unit is usually housed far from any other activity. The doctors strap you down to a small table. Then with a low rumble the table runs you into a large metal cylinder, about the length and width of a human body.

I was in the cylinder for two hours. They did let

me out a few times to give me a break, but while
inside I had to lie absolutely still, strapped down,
looking up at the top of the cylinder a few inches
above my nose. All I could think about was what
I would do in case of an earthquake. How would
I get out of there?

It took so long because at first they couldn't reg-
ister the lump on my left arm. That meant they
needed to take pictures of my right arm, in order
to compare the two. The process seemed to take
forever. When I got out I felt as though I'd been
lying in my coffin all day.

The results showed I'd been right not to feel concern. The doctors saw something abnormal, but
they thought it was what they called an "organized
hemorrhage hematoma as a result of trauma." In
short, I had ripped some muscle fiber and there
was scarring inside. A pitcher's arm is under tremendous stress, so that didn't sound too strange.

The doctors recommended that I keep an eye on
the lump, and have it examined again in six
months.

Strange to say, the house we were building in Ohio
caused us more emotion than that lump did.

As our architect sent his preliminary workups,
the costs were looking astronomical. In the short
run we could do it. I had a two-year contract with
the Giants, and every reason to think that I might
pitch for years beyond it. But when we began to
look at our situation objectively, both Janice and
I realized that it was risky. If for some reason I left
baseball, my earnings would fall to zero immediately. I'd have to get a job earning $80,000 a year

or more just to pay for the house. There aren't many such jobs available in Youngstown, Ohio. We were building a dream house that could turn into a nightmare.

It wouldn't have been our first financial nightmare, either.

Back in 1983, the year after I'd first broken into the major leagues, the Padres had offered me a three-year contract for almost three-quarters of a million dollars. That was unbelievably big money to me. Just a little more than a year before, Janice and I had been starving in the minor leagues. When I got that contract, I thought our money worries were over forever.

But they weren't. The peculiarly painful and embarrassing fact is that we managed to lose nearly all of that money.

I know the image: dumb, high-living athletes wearing big gold chains and driving expensive cars, burning up money like there's no tomorrow. But that isn't us. We managed to blow that money in a sensible, boring, middle-class way.

Modern athletes talk a lot about money. In the locker room there's more discussion of investments than squeeze plays. The smart thing is to invest, knowing that you're making a lot of money now but that your career might end tomorrow—and certainly will end while you still have a lot of life to live.

You get introduced to people who say they can offer you great investments. Every major league ballplayer seems to have a corner on a deal that will double his money in a matter of months. Like a lot of people, I got greedy. I didn't take the time to get wise counsel. I trusted my first impressions of people. I fell into a trap of talking about money with people who think they know a lot but in reality have little experience. Other players were full of talk about their investments, and soon I was too.

My biggest mistake, though, was thinking that as head of the house I should make all the financial decisions.

The fact of the matter is, Janice is the planner in our family. With her accounting background, she should have had the major input in our finances. Instead, I took over, and landed us in big trouble.

I met a financial planner who said he had a great opportunity for me. We needed a tax shelter, he said, and under his guidance we bought five condominiums—three in Arizona, two in California. I didn't ask too many questions.

We also bought a wonderful home that put us even more terrifically in debt. It was all fine, so long as my contract continued.

The three years of my contract were soon coming to an end, however, and things did not look so fine. I ended that third year with a very sore elbow. By the end of the season I couldn't pitch at all. That was the year when major league owners had colluded together not to sign free agents. Even big stars were getting no offers. When my agent began to try to negotiate a contract, the Padres acted as though they weren't interested. I began to realize that I could quite possibly be out of baseball.

When I tried to get out of the condos, I discovered that I could not give them away. They weren't worth as much as the mortgage we still owed on them.

Eventually, when things began to get scary, I sought the help and counsel of some wise friends. With their help, I began to put things right. Or, I should say, we began to put things right. The most important change was that Janice and I became partners again, in this realm as in others.

Since then, we've tried to work out our decisions together. We take the time that's required. We pray together. Together we consult people we know and can trust. It takes longer, but the results are far better.

It cost us nearly everything to get out of those condos. We also sold our San Diego dream house, to move into a smaller place. That hurt. It was embarrassing. But in the end we could look at our finances and see that we weren't in debt. We didn't have to keep pushing just to stay even. The San Diego Padres ended up offering me a one-year contract, contingent on making the team in spring training. My elbow improved and I made the team. When I was traded to San Francisco during the 1987 season, and the Giants signed me to two years guaranteed, Janice and I felt like we'd been granted a whole new beginning.

That's the context in which our dream house in Ohio became a problem to us. We were doing it again. We were building a monster house that, beautiful as it was, could put intolerable financial pressure on us.

One evening, while sitting in our for-sale home in San Diego, we began seriously discussing it. We were sprawled on the same sofa we'd been on when we'd made the decision to move home to Ohio. I was sitting up on the back this time, with my feet on the cushions.

An article Janice had been reading mentioned the importance of choosing a modest lifestyle. She asked me: "Do you think our house is modest?"

Both of us would have far preferred not to ask that question. We both wanted badly to build that house. We had a head of steam to do it. Nonetheless, we both knew the answer to her question.

"No," I said. I looked in her beautiful eyes. "There is no way in the world that house is modest."

"What are we going to do?" she asked.

I said, "Give me the phone. I'm calling the architect and we're canceling now. We're stopping the drawing."

We sold our lot and bought a smaller one. We began looking at ready-made house designs, and during spring training found one that we liked and could afford.

We entered the 1988 season without any major debts, and with the expectation that we would settle in our hometown, near the help and support of our family. That would make a huge difference in what we were about to face. We never had to agonize about the financial implications of playing or not playing baseball, and we always knew that our kids had more relatives around than they could count. However much our world got shaken, those supports were there for us to grab onto.

COMEBACK

We were certainly not anticipating any trouble in the coming year. Far from it. But looking back, it seems as though someone was anticipating for us.

Good Dreams

IF I have a dream of baseball heaven, it looks very much like spring training of 1988.

For a rookie trying to make the club, spring training is tense. But for veterans it's very relaxing. I have always had terrible springs, and 1988 was no exception. There's nothing on the line, so I don't have that fine edge competition gives. I need time to get the feeling again—the sense of balance, precision, and fluidity that comes when all the parts of my body are working in harmony. Until I get that feeling, I'm definitely hittable.

I've learned not to worry about that in the spring, however. The Giants train under the Arizona sun, and a bunch of my friends and their families rented brand-new condos together. Besides Janice and me there were Scott and Kathy Garrelts, Atlee and Jenny Hammaker, and Gary and Regina Lavelle. Gary was trying out for the Oakland A's; Atlee and Scott were my good buddies from the Giants. We all got along famously. We lived by the pool, soaking up good Arizona sun, and we treated each other's condos as our own.

In the mornings Atlee, Scott, and I would run over to the ballpark to do our work. It was all of two blocks. Sometimes our wives and kids would walk over to the ballpark to see us while we worked out. Most afternoons the team was playing a game, but if you weren't scheduled to pitch you could leave after the fifth inning. It happened I didn't make a single trip out of town for an afternoon game. We were usually drifting home to the pool by mid-afternoon.

We spent our afternoons and evenings playing together and talking together. We went out for dinner every night. Afterwards we put the kids to bed and would gather in our apartment or the Hammakers'. We stayed up late, talking over every subject in the universe, sometimes challenging each other, but nearly always learning from each other. Sometimes we'd read the Bible together. Sometimes we'd pray.

Baseball players can be a pretty lonely breed. The money you make and the media attention you receive remove you from most nonplayers who have a hard time treating you like an ordinary person. You get a lot of attention, but that's not the same as friendship. Players themselves, being constantly on the move, don't often become close. Typically, you say good-bye at the ballpark.

That's why that spring brings such wonderful memories. I don't know when I'll be together with friends like that again.

My friendship with Atlee really grew. Atlee is a very tall, long-limbed, left-handed pitcher, with a distinctively angular face that comes from a Japanese mother and an American father. We throw with the same hand, but in many other respects we're quite opposite. We were so especially when we first met. I had a lot of very strong political opinions that I wanted to tell everybody about. I saw things in black and white, right or wrong. Atlee was much more interested in people.

The word I'd use for Atlee is *sensitive.* He's very aware of his feelings. He's very aware of others' feelings. When I first met Atlee, I took a hard-line position with people. I couldn't tolerate what I considered to be stupid behavior. I thought people should see what was right, and live that way.

Atlee was different. He was truly responsive to people's needs. He was sympathetic with their weaknesses. He wasn't merely interested in what was right, he was concerned with what people felt. Consequently, he had close friends. People shared their lives with him. Atlee rubbed off on me. I wanted his friendship. I wanted to become more like him.

Still, we could tangle. Atlee wanted me to get a second opinion on the lump on my arm. He's had a lot of injuries in his career, and he's never content to take a doctor's word for things. He has to ask questions, get involved, read up on the medical literature. He wants to know as much as he possibly can before he makes a decision.

He didn't like that lump. The fact that I'd had it checked just wasn't good enough for him. He didn't believe it was a bruise or a tear. You would remember hitting something hard enough to make a bump like that, he thought.

I remember sitting out by the pool that spring, talking to him about it. The hot Arizona sun was beating down on us, and our conversation was slowly heating me up. Atlee just wouldn't accept my point of view. Finally I got good and mad. "I don't want to hear about it any more," I said. "Do you understand? I've already got a doctor. It's my arm."

Something else I've learned from Atlee: how to apologize.

He changed his direction instantly when he saw how I felt. "Hey, I'm sorry, Dave," he said. "I guess I pushed too far."

That's why we're able to disagree, to argue, even to get mad, and yet still continue as friends. I used to hold grudges. I wouldn't say anything, but I would remember. Atlee taught me how to put those things behind me.

Toward the end of spring training, when we were preparing to leave Arizona and start the season, Roger Craig came up to me at the ballpark. "Well, big boy," he drawled, "I'm going to give you the ball for opening day. You're my guy."

I was pumped up at that news. Pitching opening day is the greatest honor a manager can give you. Lots of other pitchers had done better that spring. But Roger said that I'd earned the chance with my postseason pitching in '87.

So I launched the '88 season in Dodger Stadium, going up against the great Fernando Valenzuela. The stadium was jammed. The L.A. weather was perfect. We Giants were psyched up for the season. We fully expected to win our division again, and this time to go on to the World Series.

I'll never forget my first pitch. I threw a fastball down and in to Steve Sax. He pulled out and jerked it down the line. Before I knew it, the ball had flown out of the park like a bullet. The crowd went into a frenzy. The noise seemed to press on my ears.

It wasn't a very auspicious beginning to a new season. I thought to myself, *Oh, no. Here we go!*

But then I said, "Okay, forget it. You can't change it. Let's go on from here."

I proceeded to shut the Dodgers out on two more hits the rest of the way. It seemed I'd picked up exactly where I'd left off in the playoffs. I had the feeling, that delicious sense of absolute control. We won 5–1.

You have dreams and you set goals. For all pitchers, the dream is a twenty-game winning season. I'd had that in my sights a few times. *This year,* I thought, *I'll do it.* I even told Janice when I got home for opening day in San Francisco. "You know something, baby? I think 1988 is going to be my year."

Sore Shoulder

FROM that glorious opening day I took a ride on a roller coaster. One moment I was on top and could see far into a rosy future. The next I was hurtling down, wondering if anything could ever stop my fall.

The second game I pitched was against the San Diego Padres. I had a hard time loosening up before the game. The back of my shoulder hurt. In the first inning, I gave up a two-out walk, which opened the gates for three runs to score. I only lasted four innings, and took a loss.

My third game was also against the Padres. This time I pitched well, giving up just one run in seven innings, but got no decision when the Padres hit a home run off Don Robinson in the ninth, to win 2–1.

My fourth game was also a no-decision, but it should have been a loss. I was pulled after two innings, losing 5–2. My shoulder was hurting and I couldn't work through it.

I've had almost constant soreness during my career, either in my shoulder or my elbow. Sometimes your arm starts out stiff and you just throw through the pain. Once the joints and muscles warm up they don't hurt so much. But this time the pain stayed with me.

The next game out, my fifth, I pitched well for eight innings and collected my first win since opening day.

My sixth game was against the St. Louis Cardinals. It was May 2, just one month into the season. The Cardinals must have remembered the way I'd pitched to them in the postseason, because they came into Candlestick Park hungry, ready to hit. I was absolutely terrible. My arm was killing me, and my fastball couldn't break seventy-five miles per hour. St. Louis hit me as though they were making up for last October.

I didn't last long, mercifully. After I'd survived two innings, giving up four unearned runs, Roger Craig came over in the dugout. He asked how I was doing. I admitted that my shoulder was hurting. Ordinarily I'd sooner die than admit that I wasn't able to pitch, but there was no disguising this.

I went out to start the third, but after I threw three weak balls to start the lead-off hitter, Roger took me out of the game. I went in to shower, feeling disgusted. I wanted to compete. To get beat by a batter was one thing, but to get beat by a sore shoulder was another. It was like an enemy that you couldn't see to fight. I felt helpless and frustrated.

A few days later Roger called me in to talk. Roger's office, like Roger, has an Old West theme. It's a little odd to find, tucked in a corner of the clubhouse, paintings of the Southwest desert, of horses and longhorns and Indians. Prominently displayed on one wall's dark paneling is a mounted pair of bull's horns, which I suppose could be used to poke certain players in the rear. Roger believes in motivating people. I have never needed much of that, though, and the two of us have gotten along extremely well.

I sat down, knowing approximately what news was coming. Roger kept it brief. At that moment, there was not much motivating to be done. Roger said that I was going on the fifteen-day disabled list. The coaches thought that with some rest my arm might improve.

Sore arms can and do end the career of many pitchers. I'm hypermobile, which means that my joints are extremely loose. I have the kind of build that's typical of gymnasts: big shoulders, flexible joints. Being double-jointed, I can lock my hands together behind my back and bring them all the way up over my head without breaking my grip. When I was a kid I used to pull my shoulders out of their sockets for the amusement of my friends.

This mobility may be an advantage in certain ways, but it's a disadvantage in terms of sore arms. My joints are so flexible, they wiggle around more than most people's, and they're susceptible to irritation and inflammation. I'd had a very sore shoulder in 1983, my first full season with the San Diego Padres, and missed the last six weeks of the year. At the time I made a very stupid statement. I said I hoped that from then on any soreness I got was in my elbow. During the rest of my career with San Diego, my elbow half killed me.

Now it was my shoulder again. I'd typically start warming up well, feeling fine. After three or four pitches I would try to increase my velocity. That's when I would feel a small pop, as though I'd slightly dislocated my shoulder. Immediately the pain was severe. I couldn't work through it at all, as I'd always been able to do before. I could hardly throw the ball.

Virtually the only treatment for an inflamed shoulder is rest. My fifteen days on the disabled list stretched out to twenty-five, but they were not too difficult. I was glad to skip a road trip and be around my kids. Janice was thrilled to have me home. After my initial discouragement, I took the situation in stride. I've always felt that a sore arm is part of pitching at the professional level. I'd lived through plenty of them. I expected to live through this one. The pain wouldn't kill me. I was confident that rest would bring me back.

On the 28th of May, off the disabled list, I pitched against the Philadelphia Phillies. I had nothing. I couldn't throw hard, I couldn't put the ball where I wanted it, and my slider wasn't breaking. I was, as pitchers say, throwing pus.

When you don't have your good stuff you have to pitch with your brains. I'm proud of what I did that day. In five innings I gave up two hits and one run. My arm hurt like anything, but I was able to outthink the Phillies, keeping them off balance. I'd always said that I'd know I'd arrived when I could win with lousy stuff. That day I knew. I figured I could live with the pain if I could manage to win games for the team.

Two days later we were in Montreal, and I tried to throw on the side, just warming up my arm and getting loose. The pain was so severe I almost fell down. Our pitching coach, Norm Sherry, could see that it wasn't working, and he told me to shut it down. There is a time to throw through pain, and there is a time when you're endangering your arm. Anyway, I couldn't throw through that pain no matter how much I wanted to. Nobody could.

I left the team to fly home to San Francisco. The Giants' doctor, Gordon Campbell, examined me and recommended exploratory arthroscopic surgery. Ten days later he was punching holes in me.

For some reason the preoperation procedures at Stanford Hospital were done in a huge, empty ward. Two rows of empty beds lined the room. In between was a nurse's station—with just one nurse to attend to just me. I was the only patient. I signed releases and got undressed. When everything was ready I was wheeled down to the operating room, where Dr. Campbell was waiting.

The rest I know only because I was told about it. After the anesthetist had put me under, Dr. Campbell made a small incision in the back of my shoulder—what they call a portal. Through that hole he pushed a thin, metal tube, about the diameter of a pencil. It contained an optical fiber, with a little lens on the end of it. He worked the tube up inside my shoulder, and peered into the end of it. Fluids were pumped into the joint, so that the view through the lens came to Dr. Campbell clearly—as though he were looking into a swimming pool through a snorkeling mask.

Peering into my inner workings, he found a frayed tendon where the top of the biceps muscle attaches to the shoulder. Apparently the frayed part was flopping and sticking in my shoulder joint when I flexed, and that was causing severe pain. He also found substantial scar tissue.

Portals in the back of the shoulder are only useful for looking; for actual repairs Dr. Campbell had to work from the front. He made another incision in the front of my shoulder. Inserting a little rotorooter device, Campbell went in and shaved the frayed tendon. He cleaned out scar tissue. Then he closed me up.

I woke up feeling terribly groggy from the drugs; for a long time I could hear everything going on around me, but I could not get my eyes open. When my head cleared I was nauseous. I got dressed and with Janice's help headed for home.

When we got into the car I said, "Take me to the ballpark." Atlee was pitching that afternoon, and I wanted to see the game.

Janice refused. "We're going home," she said.

"Janice, take me to Candlestick," I said.

She won. We went to our condominium. As soon as I arrived I felt awful. I lay down and fell asleep for a couple of hours of wonderful sleep.

When I woke up, I felt tremendous, and full of hope. My arm didn't even hurt. It had been routine surgery, if there is such a thing, and it was a relief to know that they'd found something they could fix. I had a lot of faith in Dr. Campbell. I was anxious to get back between the lines as soon as possible.

I began rehab with Larry Brown at the Palo Alto Sports Clinic. Larry is one of the few therapists I've known who will not baby an athlete. He knows what we're capable of doing, and he expects it of us. Larry developed a tough workout routine with weights and exercises to bring my strength back and help me overcome the surgery and the long layoff. Three days a week I'd go through the routine with him. When the team was at home I'd also go to the ballpark and work out with the guys.

Rehab therapy is extremely demanding. You work much harder than you ordinarily do during the regular season. But I like working hard, so long as I can see the goal.

Atlee and I hung around a lot together. We were like Frick and Frack. Al Rosen, the general manager of the Giants, would see us and say to Atlee, "Would you please leave that guy alone."

Atlee was on me about the lump. "Man, that lump is getting bigger than your arm!" he'd say. I wasn't thinking about it. Dr. Campbell said he had seen a lot of similar lumps on football players; they call it "blocker's bruise." My feeling was that if the doctor wasn't worried, then I shouldn't be either. I was much more concerned about my shoulder.

Despite the operation, and despite all my hard work, my shoulder didn't seem to be getting any better. I was throwing the ball, but it still hurt.

When you're sitting on the sidelines, it's very easy to lose perspective. You get depressed. You think the worst. I began to wonder whether my days in baseball were over.

Part of me felt ready for that. I was knocking myself out every day and seeing no improvement. I wasn't getting the joy of playing the game.

I talked to Atlee about it one day, while I was riding the stationary bike in the Giants' weight room. It's an open room full of exercise machines and weights. I spend a lot of time in it, getting my work in. For me it's a quiet, relaxing place.

Atlee was in a philosophic mood. He said, "We take so much for granted in this game. We assume that we're going to come back from injury, but you know, our careers could be over now and we don't even know it."

It surprised him, I think, when I told him I was prepared for that. "When I leave this," I said, "I won't look back. I'd like to get my ten years in so I'll be fully vested in the pension. After that, I'll walk away from it and be perfectly happy."

We got in an argument. Atlee had watched one of his closest friends struggle through the process of leaving baseball. He described how this friend would feel every February, when spring training began and he felt lost and uncertain of his life's purpose. "There's no way," Atlee said, "that you can walk away from baseball and not be affected. You've been playing since you were a little kid. It's going to be a lot harder than you think it is."

Soon we were shouting at each other. "Don't tell me what I'm feeling," I said. "You don't know what's inside me. I know I won't miss it."

Atlee said, "I know you will. It's a part of us."

Field of Dreams

IN the movie *Field of Dreams* a young farmer in
Iowa hears a mysterious voice, telling him that
he's supposed to build a baseball diamond in the
middle of his cornfield. His neighbors think he's
crazy, but he builds the diamond anyway. He has
no idea what the purpose is. He just waits to find
out. He's sure there's a reason.

What happens is even stranger than the voice
out of nowhere. "Shoeless Joe" Jackson appears.
A great player of the past, Jackson was banned
from professional baseball because of a gambling
scandal. He died in anonymity and disgrace. Now
he appears, coming out of some otherworldly ex-
istence. He wants to play baseball. The diamond
is meant for him.

Soon he recruits a whole team of ballplayers out
of the otherworldly realm. They appear every day
in their old-time uniforms, play together, and then
disappear back where they've come from, through
the cornfield beyond center field.

Once, as one of them vanishes, he cries out in
a joking imitation of the *Wizard of Oz*'s Wicked
Witch: "Help me! I'm melting!"

Melting away—that's how the thought of leaving baseball sounds to those of us who have been fortunate enough to play. What other career takes you to such a pinnacle of success and then ends by the age of forty? Here for a few years we play a boy's game, on a beautiful green field before fans who love us. We give it all our passionate attention, and baseball seems, like all boyhood games, as though it could last forever. It's the only life we know. We've never held a real job. We can't imagine what's beyond. We just can't picture life without baseball. When we leave the game, will we melt away?

By August, after much hard work, my arm strength was back. The Giants' season had not gone as well as we had hoped, but the Dodgers and the Reds were stumbling badly, and we still had a shot at the pennant. The team's management hoped to get me back in the pitching rotation for the stretch drive. They decided it was time for me to do my twenty-day rehabilitation assignment in the minor leagues. This would be the last stage before they reactivated me on the big-league team.

I was sent down to our Triple-A team in Phoenix, where I started against the Colorado Springs Sox, the Cleveland Indians' Triple-A farm team. I started the game with high hopes, which lasted less than an hour. I got shellacked. My arm was still killing me, and I couldn't have broken a pane of glass with my fastball. The speed gun registered my fastest pitch at seventy-eight miles per hour, which will definitely not get you a contract coming out of high school. I lasted two and two-thirds innings, giving up eleven hits and five runs.

COMEBACK

Norm Sherry, our pitching coach, had come down to Phoenix with me. He strolled slowly out to the mound and asked me what was up. When I told him how I felt he said, "Shut it down." The next day I flew back to San Francisco. There wasn't any point in trying to pitch with that kind of pain.

I stayed with the team, feeling pretty low. The whole team was falling into a dismal state by then. By the end of the summer we had dropped out of contention. Everybody was putting in their time, and thinking about clearing out for home.

I hate to give up. *Maybe,* I kept thinking, *I can work through this pain.* I decided to try pitching batting practice. I simply couldn't do it.

Then I tried just throwing the ball, playing catch. But my shoulder hurt so much I couldn't stand it. I obviously wasn't going to pitch again in 1988. The whole season was a loss for me.

As Dr. Campbell explained it to me, once a shoulder like mine gets aggravated, the problems tend to come back again and again. He said there was not much they could do for me, except wait and see how the shoulder responded to rest. If that didn't work, there was one drastic possibility. Some outfielders had tried a surgical procedure in which their shoulder muscles were shortened, in order to tighten their joints. The procedure was quite experimental, and had never been tried on a pitcher. We discussed it as a last-ditch possibility, which probably says less about the viability of such a procedure than it does about how bleak things were looking for me.

*　　　*　　　*

By September, Janice had left with the kids for Ohio. We wanted to get them settled in school. Our little place south of San Francisco was pretty lonely without my family. I wasn't doing a thing with the team, just riding the stationary bike to keep my legs in shape. I couldn't touch a baseball without wincing. I finally approached Roger Craig and Al Rosen, our general manager, to ask them whether I could go home to be with my family. They said sure. So I packed up.

Before leaving I talked with Dr. Campbell about getting another MRI done on my lump. It was just routine. A little over six months had passed since I'd had the first one, and six months was the time period the doctors in San Diego had recommended before I got it checked again.

By then the lump was clearly visible. It stood out on the side of my arm like half a golf ball, and nearly as hard as one, too. Mark Letendre, our trainer, thought it looked bigger simply because my arm muscles had atrophied with the inactivity of lying around. I normally have beefy arms and shoulders, and they'd certainly shrunk. To me, though, the lump looked bigger. Atlee was sure it was bigger.

They did the MRI on September 9, and the next day I flew home. It was a bittersweet feeling to leave. I'd played very little baseball during the year, and my arm troubles had certainly contributed to the team's problems. It's lousy to feel that you've been well paid for doing absolutely nothing of worth to anyone. I couldn't help my performance, but I still felt bad about it. Naturally, I compared my feelings with the excitement I'd had at the start of the season. I'd expected this to be my year.

It was great, though, to get out of the airplane into the crisp fall air of Ohio, to see the leaves beginning to turn, to hug my kids and my wife, and to be greeted by my family and friends from my boyhood town. I was still something special in Boardman, Ohio.

Our new home was under construction, and one of the first things I did was go see it. The workmen were all over it, doing finish work. The exterior was done; I stood on the front lawn and felt a terrific sense of pride looking at it. Walking through the bare rooms, I got a sense of what it would be like to live there. I could hardly wait to move in. In the meantime we were living with my parents.

A few days after I returned home I got a call from Dr. Campbell. I wasn't surprised to hear from him. I'd expected he'd let me know the results of the MRI.

He talked in his gentle, businesslike voice. "Dave, there's a soft tissue mass on the end of your deltoid muscle," he said. "I've had some specialists look at the film, and they aren't sure what it is. It could be nothing, but I'd recommend you go see a doctor in your area."

He asked me who I knew in the area, and I told him that we lived about an hour's drive from the Cleveland Clinic. He said that was great. He knew a Dr. Bergfeld there, the team doctor for the Cleveland Indians. He said he'd get me an appointment with him.

*　　*　　*

The next day found Janice and me in a little medical examining room at the Cleveland Clinic, waiting to be seen. I was sitting on the examining table, Janice in a chair. A parade of medical people preceded Dr. Bergfeld.

Neither Janice nor I was particularly concerned. For us this was just a routine check on a minor problem.

We were struck by the fanfare for Dr. Bergfeld. We'd never heard of him, but evidently he was somebody special. It was as though an entourage were preparing the way for a king. We would see the man himself only after we had been thoroughly checked by other, lesser figures.

One doctor asked me a lot of questions, took down my medical history, inquired about other injuries, how long I'd played baseball, and so on. When he was gone another group came in. They had me take my shirt off. They looked at my arm, felt it, rotated it.

We began to wonder whether we would ever see Dr. Bergfeld. Janice and I were talking quietly together when we heard the cadre of doctors shuffling around outside the door. Apparently Dr. Bergfeld had arrived. The film from the MRI had been sent out from California, and we heard it flap into position as they stuck it up over the lights. In low tones the doctors were discussing what they saw. Then we heard the distinct words from one deep voice, rising over the others. "Look at that tumor."

Until that very moment, no such possibility had crossed my mind, or Janice's either. I had thought we were there to have some scar tissue checked.

We were just making sure everything was okay, just being careful.

When we heard the word "tumor," it was as though the entire floor fell away and left us standing on a tiny chunk of safe ground hundreds of feet above a deep crevasse. Life that had seemed so safe and predictable only moments before was now revealed to be at the verge of calamity.

I looked at Janice. She looked at me. I could see from her eyes that she was shocked and scared. But she's a strong person, and she initiated the right response. "I think we better pray," she said.

"Yeah," I said. "We better pray right now."

I got off the examining table and sat on a chair beside her. We held hands. It wasn't a long prayer.

"Dear God," I said, "we don't know what's happening. We don't know what this means. Help us to get through it, no matter what is involved. Help us to face whatever comes."

We didn't pray for long, because Dr. Bergfeld was coming in.

Preparing for the Worst, Hoping for the Best

DR. John Bergfeld came into the examining room, followed by his entourage. By the time everybody had crowded in, we made quite a little group.

I felt at home with Dr. Bergfeld right away. I can't think of anybody I'd rather meet just moments after hearing the word "tumor." He is a tall, confident man, with an exuberant manner. He has a way of making you feel that everything is in competent hands, that everything will be okay.

We needed all the reassurance we could get. I was stunned. I couldn't take in what was happening to me. Janice was scared. She wanted details.

Dr. Bergfeld took my arm, moved it around, examined it. He asked a few questions. He told me right away, "Dave, this may be a tumor. We definitely need to do a biopsy on this. I'm going to send you up to see an oncologist."

When he said "oncologist," my heart skipped a beat. I knew that an oncologist is a cancer doctor.

He kept talking calmly, though, as if we were discussing the weather. "David, I don't think this is a malignant tumor. You've had it for over a year now and the rate of growth is much slower than we would normally expect for a malignancy."

"But," he said, "we need to be sure of that. So I want to send you up to see Dr. Muschler."

At Dr. Bergfeld's instructions, one of the doctors in his entourage led me to the elevator and down to the x-ray room, moving me past everybody who was waiting. They had me hold my breath at various angles, and shot the pictures. Afterwards Dr. Bergfeld escorted Janice and me up to the fifth floor to meet Dr. Muschler.

We shook hands in the hallway outside the examining rooms. I thought, *Man, this guy's hot off the presses.* He had wire-rim glasses, and looked young enough to be taking his first college biology class. This was the doctor?

For what seemed to be the thirtieth time that day my arm got examined. Dr. Muschler explored the flesh beneath the skin, moving my arm into various positions, touching that golf-ball-sized lump. Finally he looked at me and said, "I recommend you have a biopsy on this. I don't think"—here he sounded just like Bergfeld—"I don't think we're dealing with a malignant tumor. But we can't be sure."

I wanted to jump out of my skin and say, "What do you mean you can't be sure? You're talking about my life!"

But he had a very reassuring way of talking. "We could really very well be dealing with scar tissue," he said. But he didn't think that was it. "I think we're probably dealing with a fibrous tumor."

Janice responded in her typical, responsible way. While I went off into deep space, she asked questions. She was astonished that Dr. Muschler could discuss a tumor so calmly—as though it were an ordinary event. Of course in his medical world, it is.

I asked him when he wanted to do the biopsy. He said, "As soon as possible."

Janice and I should have had a lot to talk about on our drive home, but I found it hard to know what to say. I didn't even quite know what I was feeling. All the ordinary chitchat seemed too commonplace.

Janice was in shock too. She is very rarely at a loss for words, but she was then. Every time she would start to talk she stopped short. What could she say?

So we drove down the highway, each of us in a separate world of our own thoughts.

In a sense not much had happened. A few doctors had poked and prodded me, and they'd ordered up some more tests. I kept thinking of those words, "We can't be sure." We didn't know a thing more than when we'd walked into the clinic an hour or so earlier. But our world had been turned inside out. So had our minds.

When we got to my parents' home we didn't know just what to tell them, either. Obviously they were upset at the news, but they didn't ask too many questions. They always try to take an optimistic view of things. It was easier for them not to know too much, I suspect. Of course we all hoped it would turn out to be nothing serious. We didn't tell Tiffany and Jonathan.

The biopsy was done two days later. I asked for permission to stay awake through the operation, because I'd hoped to see what they were doing. But they draped a sheet in front of me, so I might as well have been asleep. The operation itself was a very strange sensation. My arm was completely numb from the anesthetic, but I felt them pulling on me—tugging to get a piece of the tumor out through the incision. It didn't take long, maybe half an hour.

After some recovery time, Dr. Muschler came in to talk to Janice and me. They had given me something to help me relax, so I felt very slow-witted. That was all right, since I counted on Janice to handle the questions.

Muschler seemed optimistic as he described the tumor's position. It was growing on the base of the deltoid muscle, near where it attaches to the humerus bone. He drew a picture to show us. The deltoid is the large, shield-shaped muscle that wraps over the top of your shoulder. It starts broad at the top and narrows to a point where it's attached to the middle of the humerus, which is the large bone between your shoulder and your elbow. Dr. Muschler said the tumor had stretched fingers up from that attachment into the muscle. He said he couldn't be sure without the lab results, but the tumor looked like what he had thought: a fibrous tumor. He was reasonably certain that it wasn't a life-threatening malignancy. "But I can't be one hundred percent sure," he said.

I didn't find that as reassuring as he meant it to be. My mind kept zeroing in on one phrase. I heard it again and again in my mind: "We can't be sure." I had a tumor in my body, something that was not me, an organism that might be death growing within. The doctor didn't think it would kill me, but he also admitted that he couldn't be sure. On topics of life and death, one percent of doubt is a very large amount.

Janice went home feeling encouraged. For her, it was enough that the doctor thought the risk seemed very low. For me, the same information produced a very different set of reactions. You can't be objective about your own life—at least, I can't.

To make a comparison, I know that skydiving is a very safe sport, if conducted with the proper precautions. If I meet a skydiver about to go up to dive, I'll treat it pretty casually. The possibility of his death will not seem that great to me.

Yet my feelings will change very dramatically if I am up in a small plane minding my own business when the pilot suddenly breaks into a sweat, says we are in trouble, and tells me to get my parachute on. Then the safe nature of skydiving will seem far, far away. When Dr. Muschler said he couldn't be one hundred percent sure, I felt like I was standing in the doorway of the plane, about to be pushed out.

With part of my mind I was very objective. The doctors would treat the lump, it would go away, and I would go on with life. Another part of my mind, though, couldn't stop thinking that I might die, leaving my wife and children behind.

As we were leaving the hospital, one of Dr. Muschler's assistants pulled me aside and gave me his card.

"You know, I used to play professional football

for the Cincinnati Bengals," he said. "When I left
that, it was really difficult for me. If you need to
talk to somebody over the next few months, give
me a call and we can get together for dinner.
Maybe I can help you through this transition."

After we left, Janice looked at me with a puzzled
expression. "David, why did he say that?"

I didn't know. I was thinking that the tumor
might end my life, if it were the wrong kind. I
hadn't considered the possibility that even if it
were the right kind, it could end my career. It was,
after all, still a painless little lump.

The days following the biopsy were quiet ones, full
of intense concentration for me. The baseball season had ended and the playoffs were about to
begin, but I was living in a world far removed from
that.

I didn't have much to say. Janice didn't guess
what I was feeling, and I didn't know how to explain it to her. I was quiet. I sat and filled my eyes
with my wife and my children. I couldn't get
enough of being near them.

It was an anxious time, waiting, just waiting to
hear the news. When the phone rang I always
wondered whether it would be the results.

Yet it was a good kind of anxiety, if I can put
it that way. Just looking at Janice reminded me
how much I loved her, of how much she did for me.
I stared at her and I stared at my kids, thinking
they were the most beautiful sight in the entire universe. Some nights when Tiffany and Jonathan
were asleep I would go into their room and listen
to them slowly breathing. I thought of how often

I didn't have time for them. On so many occasions, when they had asked me to play ball, I'd told them, "I'm busy reading right now; give me ten minutes"—and then the phone would ring and I never would get to play with them. During those days of waiting I did play ball, or whatever else they wanted to play.

I also thought about my eternal destination. I felt a deep sense of security there—that if I were going to die, I knew what would come next. That meant a lot to me.

I don't ordinarily think much about heaven and hell. I'm too busy keeping up with the day-to-day concerns of life. But in those days I found that my perspective shifted. Some things that mattered a lot in the day-to-day routine of living mattered much less. Some things that I seldom considered mattered a great deal more.

Janice's mother had died a few years before, during my first summer in the major leagues. Her death had made a similar impact, shifting my perspective.

Janice's mother had hated to fly, so she hadn't come out to the West Coast to see me pitch. She got her first chance to cheer for me as a major leaguer when we were playing a double header in Cincinnati. A whole host of my family and friends had driven up from Youngstown. Janice's mother was among them.

At that time I was in the bull pen, so I couldn't be sure I'd get in a game. But sure enough, in the seventh inning of the first game I got the call to warm up. From the bull pen, while I was getting ready, I noticed a commotion in the stands. I pointed it out to Terry Kennedy, my catcher. "Man, I sure hope whoever it is up there is okay," I said.

Later my dad told me what had happened. Janice's mother, noticing that I was warming up, had asked my dad whether I was likely to be called on. Moments later she had fallen backwards in her seat. She had died immediately from a heart attack.

But no one told me. I came into the game and pitched, we took our break between games, and then we played the second game. Still no one told me, though people in the dugout knew. They had me warming up in the bull pen, though I didn't go in. After the game the pitching coach called me into a private room in the clubhouse and quietly told me the bad news: Janice's mother had been the person in the stands.

My only thought was to call Janice, who had stayed behind in San Diego with our baby Tiffany. Janice and her mother were extremely close. I knew that the news would half kill her.

I didn't think until later about how strange it was that no one had told me. Apparently the game had to go on, regardless of my mother-in-law's death. To me, though, the game didn't seem very important under those circumstances. No game can matter much when you're looking at death. Nothing matters, except love.

Love, not baseball, is what I thought about during those few days of anxiety after the biopsy. Sometimes in the mornings, after Janice had gotten up with the kids, I would lie in the basement, where we were sleeping, and think how much I loved her. I thought how much I loved Tiffany and Jonathan.

One thought did not enter my mind. I never thought, *Why me?* I didn't feel sorry for myself. I wasn't wondering why God had treated me so unfairly. I wasn't feeling as though God was mean and vindictive.

I know that those thoughts do come to people who are facing cancer, because many people have asked me about them. Some have been convinced that I must be thinking that way. For many people it seems a battle with cancer is also a battle with bitterness.

I don't claim any credit for myself, but I didn't think that way. Janice didn't either. It just wasn't in our mindset. God had put us through some experiences and taught us some lessons that prepared us to face the worst. To explain it to you, I'd have to take you back to my minor league days in places like Amarillo, Texas, and Colombia, South America, and tell you what it was like on our way to the show, the big time.

In Barranquilla and Amarillo

I realize that many people switch off when an athlete starts talking about God. They feel that such talk cheapens the very personal issue of faith.

To some extent I share that reaction. Some athletes use God like a trinket. They think that if they can latch on to God, they're going to go four for four, or they're going to hit a home run in the bottom of the ninth inning and win the ball game. Consequently they show up for chapel services before a Sunday ball game. They think, *If I'm there and God sees me, he might honor my game today.*

That is bogus religion. It really shows a gigantic disrespect for God. Any genuine God of the universe must be a lot bigger than my desire to increase my batting average. If that's all God is to somebody, then God is just a superstition.

Maybe I feel so strongly about this because it's not too far from the image of God I once had.

I grew up in a devout Catholic home, and I always tried to practice my faith. To me that meant attending church once a week. Sunday morning was the time slot for respecting God.

During the baseball season, going to church on

Sunday wasn't easy. When I was in the minor leagues I began going to baseball chapel. Baseball chapel is a brief, voluntary meeting held at the ballpark on Sunday before the game. I went so regularly that in Buffalo, New York, I became the chapel leader.

I was playing for the Buffalo Bisons, the Double-A farm team for the Pittsburgh Pirates. Double-A is the midpoint in the minor leagues. Triple-A is above it, the last rung on the ladder to the major leagues. A-level ball is below it, the first call for kids just out of school. Double-A is definitely not a glamorous life. Very few of the players will ever make the major leagues. The crowds are small. The stadiums tend to be old and dilapidated. In Buffalo, for example, the stadium was crawling with rats, who feasted on peanuts and popcorn under the stands.

We usually had guest speakers for chapel, and I heard a lot about God from them. Many of them gave testimonies about a personal relationship with God. But that kind of talk didn't really click for me.

I didn't really need God. I'd always depended on my own abilities and my own drive, and I'd done pretty well with that. I thought of myself as a decent person. God received his due on Sunday morning. The rest of my life belonged to me.

In the fall of 1979, after my first year at Buffalo, I was asked by the Pirates, who "owned" me, to play winter ball in Colombia, South America. They asked me, but I didn't really think I had much of a choice. I was not a bonus baby who had been signed for big money because he had a big future. In fact, I'd been told repeatedly that I'd never make it to the big leagues.

It had always been that way. Out of high school I hadn't gotten a scholarship to play baseball at a big name school, so I'd attended Youngstown State University, my hometown college. Youngstown is definitely not where major league scouts hang out. I had my big chance at the end of my junior year, when about thirty scouts came to a postseason playoff game I was pitching at Southern Illinois University. At the time my record was 7–1, with an earned run average of 0.88, leading all college Division II pitchers. Unfortunately, I got bombed that day—really bombed. We lost 26 to 1. Nobody offered me a contract. Nobody even spoke to me.

The next year, as a senior, my record wasn't nearly as good. I was invited to a couple of tryouts, and one scout for the Pittsburgh Pirates showed some interest. He said he didn't know whether I'd get chosen, but he'd see what he could do. I was drafted by the Pirates in the twenty-first round. They offered me no money, just a chance to play. I was definitely not on the top of the Pirates' list as a potential big league player.

So when the organization suggested I go to Colombia, I wasn't about to argue. As a matter of fact, Janice and I were excited about going. We were two kids, married for one year, who had hardly been out of the Midwest. Now we were being sent to Barranquilla, a coastal city facing north on the Caribbean. We had visions of tropical beaches and exotic Latin nights. That sounded considerably better than a winter in Youngstown, Ohio.

We were totally unprepared to confront the Third World. At the airport, we saw automatic weapons everywhere. Not long after we arrived, team officials called in all the American players and warned us never to do drugs. They said that were we arrested in Colombia, no one would be able to help us. The maximum sentence, someone told us, was ten years—because no one had ever lived more than ten years in a Colombian jail.

We saw open sewers around our apartment in an old high rise in the center of town. The poverty we encountered as we walked down our street made us sick. So did the filth. Rather than a tropical paradise, we were in a grimy, industrial city. It was unbearably sticky and hot, and Janice got horribly sick. Our tiny, one-bedroom apartment had old gray tile and awful red leather furniture. The cockroaches were as big as mice. Next door were five guys in a two-bedroom apartment who were sick all the time; their bathroom vented into our bedroom, and you can imagine how it smelled.

Most Americans were sick. You couldn't drink the water, and the food wasn't to our liking. Our team was allowed seven American ballplayers. We stuck close together for mutual comfort.

When we played a night game, they'd shut off electricity for half the city in order to get power to light the stadium. If you played poorly—and I did—people would throw corncobs at you. Fans figured out that Janice was my wife—she was the only blond in the stands—and would hiss at her and make signs with their hands like a gun pointed at her head.

It sounds funny, but it wasn't. We were there for two months, the worst two months of our lives. I got sick with a 104-degree fever. I was out of my head for days. Janice would try to keep cold compresses under my arms and on my legs while I thrashed around in a delirium. She would lie on top of me, trying to hold me down, and pray that somehow God would help us.

We did pray, out of desperation. We talked about God far more than we ever had. But he was strictly a generic God, far away from us, vague and unknown. We needed help, and he was the last possible source of it.

I lost fifteen pounds in five days from the fever, and when I tried to come back and pitch I was so weak I had nothing on the ball. The team released me. Nobody could have convinced me I'd ever be happy to be released from a team. But when I got the news, I thought I was the luckiest guy in Colombia.

The timing was great, just before Christmas. Janice and I could barely wait to get out of that country. It seemed too good to be true: We would be home for the holidays.

Then we got to the airport with all our luggage and discovered that the team's owner hadn't taken care of our visas properly. We weren't being allowed out of the country. The uniformed officials suggested that because of the holidays it would take two weeks to get the papers straightened out.

Janice began to cry. She was scared.

We took our luggage back to our apartment, feeling helpless and afraid. We wanted so badly to get out of that country, to get home, to be on familiar ground again. We were desperate, ready to try almost anything.

The next day the team's owner walked us through customs with money ready to pay off anybody who recognized us. He had done something to our visas, and we had to lie about what we had been doing in Colombia. We got through, fortunately. If we had been caught we might still be there.

When we got home I promised Janice that we would never go back to Colombia again. The Pirates sent me to play another year of Double-A ball in Buffalo, and I had a good year, thirteen wins and seven losses. I hoped to advance to Triple-A ball.

The key in the minor leagues is to keep moving upward. If you stay at one level too long, you'll be released. Too many other players are pushing upward, and they want your slot.

But once again, the Pirates "suggested" that I play winter ball in Colombia. They said I didn't have to go, but that if I had aspirations of reaching the big leagues they recommended it strongly. Under the circumstances I didn't feel that I had any choice. It was either go or forget about my future in baseball. So I broke my promise to Janice. She was really upset. She could see my point of view, but the memory of Colombia was too strong for her. She couldn't stand it again.

We decided she should stay home and wait for me. She got a good job with an accounting firm in

Sarasota, Florida. We needed the money, because I made only $600 or $700 a month playing baseball. I went back to Barranquilla—to the same apartment, in fact—without her.

If anything it was worse. I missed her like crazy. There were nights I got down on my hands and knees to beg God for help, because I felt so scared and alone.

Janice and I first met in high school, when we were both dating somebody else. When we double-dated to the drive-in movies, Janice refused to sneak in. Consequently, I went in with her, since I had the car. The others were going to walk in through a hole in the fence.

While we were alone, I took one good look at her and said, "Someday, baby, you and I are going to be together for real."

It took a while for my prediction to come true. I was attracted to her as the best-looking girl I'd seen. I wanted her for my own, but for a long time she wasn't willing to go out with me. I figured persistence would win out. I was right. We got married after college, as soon as I could earn the semblance of a living that baseball offered.

By that winter in Colombia we'd been married for two years, and I hardly knew how to live without her. I depend on her for friendship. I depend on her for wisdom, too—she has a very deep, careful way of thinking things through, which balances my sometimes impetuous nature. I just plain like her. I always want to be with her. Always.

With her so far away, the only solace I had was from a small bunch of players who were Christians and used to get together for fellowship. I'd sit in with them, not from any great conviction that I belonged, but just because I needed somebody to be with. Again I was exposed to a lot of conversation about God. I certainly didn't buy it all, but I didn't reject it either. I guess I considered it like a college bull session, where guys trade opinions.

I pitched terribly, got released again, and left Colombia to join Janice in Sarasota. That was where the Pirates held spring training.

I came away from Colombia a subtly different person. I was no longer so sure of my ability to make life work in my favor. I'd found some things were beyond my control. I'd called out to God for help, in a sense suggesting—though I could not have put this in words—that perhaps he deserved more than respect one hour a week. My image of him was ripe for change.

I felt I'd reached the do-or-die stage of my baseball career. I had to make the jump to Triple-A.

Unfortunately, by the time we were down to our last spring games, we had nineteen pitchers on our Triple-A roster. They were going to keep nine, and seven of my competitors had pitched in the major leagues.

I have always used adversity in my favor. For example, I'd heard through the grapevine that Murray Cook, the Pirates' farm system director, had said I'd never make it as a big league starter. Hearing that didn't slow me down. Just the opposite. I used it to motivate myself. I drove myself to prove him wrong. I looked forward to looking him in the eye after I'd started my first game with the Pittsburgh Pirates.

I'm a realist, however. I could see that my chances of making this Triple-A club were close to zero. And I couldn't see going back to Double-A for the third straight year.

The Pirates probably couldn't see that either. It was either play me at Triple-A, trade me, or release me. I thought the chances were pretty good that I would be released. That would be the end of my baseball career—not a pretty thought.

That spring I sat in a bull session with a bunch of guys talking about which ball club would be the best to play for. The consensus was that the San Diego Padres would be ideal, because they had a great organization, the future of the team looked bright, and San Diego was a wonderful city. Also, the Padres' Triple-A team was in Hawaii. Even if you didn't make it to the big leagues, you'd get to play in Hawaii.

A few days after that discussion, as spring training was winding up, Murray Cook called for me in the clubhouse. At that time of year, when the farm director calls your name your heart starts thumping. All the guys were diving into their lockers, laughing and pretending to hide from Cook. They began yelling, "You're out of here, Dravecky! You're gone!"

Murray looked at me and said, "We've traded you, Dave."

Given the situation, that wasn't bad news. In the back of my mind I was immediately thinking, *Gosh, we were just talking about San Diego the other day. I hope he says San Diego.*

Sure enough, he said San Diego. Immediately I was thinking, *Say Hawaii, please say Hawaii!*

But instead he said, "We've traded you to San Diego, and you're going to Amarillo."

Where on earth was Amarillo? I knew for sure it wasn't in Hawaii. When I talked around to the other guys, they said that Amarillo, Texas, was the worst possible place to play: hot, windy, flat, and dull. Somebody said if he were given the choice of playing in Amarillo or hell, he would choose hell. Amarillo was a Double-A team, too—my third year at that level.

But I thought, *Oh well, at least I'm with a new club and I have a new chance to prove myself.* I went to Amarillo, leaving Janice behind to complete the tax season. She needed to earn money for us to live on during the coming year.

In Amarillo I checked into the Holiday Inn, where the ballplayers were staying until we found other accommodations. The room was the same one we've all slept in: two beds and a shag carpet. My roommate had already arrived but he wasn't in the room. I left and met some of the other players, then returned to the room and found him waiting.

His name was Byron Ballard. He had brilliant red hair and freckles; he was tall with size fifteen feet. I liked the guy immediately. Everybody did. He seemed incredibly joyful about life. He had a wonderful, zany sense of humor.

I saw some literature lying on his bed, Christian literature associated with baseball chapel. I commented on it and he asked me whether I was familiar with baseball chapel.

"I sure am," I said. "I was the chapel leader in Buffalo."

I saw Byron's eyes light up. He immediately assumed I was a born-again Christian, and made some kind of reference to that. I realized I needed to straighten him out. "I'm sorry," I said, "but there's no way. I really don't understand that terminology at all."

I suppose most people would have taken that as a rebuff, but Byron didn't. He kept talking to me. More than that, he got out a Bible and showed me where Jesus talked about being born again. (It's in John 3:3.) I was impressed. The guy obviously knew something.

During the next weeks, we talked again, and again, and again. Byron was not a guy to ram something down my throat. On the contrary, I was asking him questions. Because of Colombia, I was open to rethinking my life.

I already knew that there was a God, I considered myself a Christian, and I believed that the Bible was God's Word. I got all that from my upbringing. But I had never read the Bible. Once, when we were first married, Janice had suggested we read it together. Something in her church upbringing had given her the idea that it would be a good thing for a married couple to do. But I had said no way. "I can never read that thing, Janice. It doesn't even make sense. It's for the priests to read, not me. If you want to read it, that's your business, but don't ask me to do it with you."

Byron didn't tell me his answers to my questions. He showed me answers in the Bible. For me that was very important, because I had no doubts that the Bible was true. I soon found out, through reading with Byron, that the Bible contained plenty of very understandable material. It gave me a perspective on God that turned my religious ideas upside down. God wasn't distant and vague in the Bible. He was active and close to people. God had come to earth as Jesus, who was visible, personal, concerned about people like me—who had, in fact, died for people like me.

But I had a lot of questions. I felt I was basically a good person. I had difficulty understanding why Byron thought I was a sinner. I knew that I wasn't perfect, but did that make me a sinner?

Byron showed me where the Bible says that all human beings are sinners, because all fall short of the glory God intended them to have. (That's in Romans 3:23.) I was amazed. I couldn't understand why no one had told me this before.

My next question was: How do I get rid of my sin? Byron again showed me places in the Bible that describe the need to turn away from your sin in repentance—to confess that you're a sinner, and ask God to forgive you because of what Jesus did on the cross. One of these Bible verses has become a kind of theme for me: Romans 10:9. It reads like this: "If you confess with your mouth, 'Jesus is Lord,' and believe in your heart that God raised him from the dead, you will be saved."

I didn't become a believer overnight. I watched Byron like a hawk. And that drew me. It wasn't what he said that convinced me so much as the way he lived. In every situation he was the same: full of joy, brimming over with love for this God he talked about. I kept calling Janice and pumping her with the stuff I was learning. I told her that I'd met the greatest guy, who was showing me all kinds of amazing stuff in the Bible. She couldn't believe what she was hearing. She was horrified. She thought I was getting hooked into some cult. She told me, "All I ask is that you don't do anything until I get there."

So I didn't. I wanted to make a commitment, but I respected Janice so much that I was willing to wait. It was two full months before she could join me. By then my teammates were sick of hearing me talk about her.

Janice arrived with a whole different set of questions than I had. She'd been struggling with them ever since she'd left Colombia.

Colombia had made me feel for the first time in my life that I truly needed God. For Janice, it had the opposite effect: It created doubt that God even existed. She'd grown up believing in a God who was benignly taking care of the world, like a white-haired grandfather. That didn't square with the injustice she saw all around in Colombia—the hunger, the poverty, the hopelessness. So she'd concluded there must not be any grandfather-God.

She'd been deeply depressed, though I hadn't known it. We didn't communicate very well then, even though we were crazy about each other. She'd become depressed because her simple, happy view of the world had been blown to bits.

When Janice came to Amarillo, she felt really nervous about me. She was afraid her baseball-playing husband was being changed into a religious fanatic. The last thing she wanted to hear about was God. That was all I wanted to talk about. As usual I wasn't very patient with her. I kept wanting her to see things the way I did, and to move ahead as fast as I was moving. But we did love each other, and with the help of other people and a few books she began sorting through her questions. I saw her gradually grow excited with me.

We could see that if God was as personal as Byron—and the Bible—said, our basic orientation would have to change. If God truly cared about every detail of life, we couldn't any longer assume that we knew what was best for ourselves, adding on God as an afterthought. Vague, generic gods you can treat any way you like. But a personal God requires commitment.

Eventually we made a decision. We committed ourselves together to follow the personal God we learned about in the Bible, to follow Jesus wherever he might lead us. We admitted to him that we needed to be forgiven if we were going to be regarded as his children, because we fell short of him in a million ways. We chose to believe what the Bible said: that Jesus Christ had died on the cross precisely because of that sinfulness, to take it away. We accepted his death as given on our behalf, and promised to live our lives in his love from that time on, with his help.

God is personal. That lesson, learned in Amarillo, changed our lives forever. It transformed our response to the news we heard seven years later at the Cleveland Clinic.

It prevented us from responding to the tumor with bitterness and anger. If I'd still had an image of God as a distant Keeper of the Rules, then it would have seemed very unfair to me that I was getting a tougher deal than a lot of other ballplayers. What was happening wasn't fair, and a Rulekeeper God either didn't exist, or I had good reason for being very angry at him.

But that's not my image of God any longer. He's not the Cosmic Bookkeeper, the one to blame if things don't work out the way you think they should. Life isn't always fair, at least in the short run, but the Bible taught me not to confuse life with God. When you're confronted with trouble you don't ask, "Why me?" You ask God, "What do you want me to do in this situation?"

Because the God who revealed himself as Jesus is full of love. He never deserts his children. Janice and I entered this difficult period, when life was often beyond our control, with a deep conviction that God was for us. Jesus had given his life for us. There was nothing else—no other good thing—he would withhold. We expected to see God's love in whatever came—however strange the twists and turns of the road might be. That fundamental belief gave us a deep well of hope to draw from.

Making It to the Big Leagues

FROM one point of view, Amarillo was as bad as I'd heard. The heat was blistering, the wind whipped over a treeless prairie, and tumbleweeds were about the only thing shaking on Saturday night. Our stadium was located next to the stock-yards, which provided epidemic flies. When the wind came from that direction you didn't feel like breathing, the smell was so awful.

Yet the year we spent in Amarillo was the most important in our lives—and the most wonderful. We weren't in a glamorous town. We didn't have any money. Janice and I shared our apartment with a teammate, a single guy named Mike Barba, just to split the rent. But I will always remember the closeness we had with a bunch of players and their wives there. We were all new Christians, very excited about learning together. The group of us attended Pastor Roy Wheeler's Paramount Terrace Christian Church. We spent hours reading the Bible and discussing it and calling people up to ask questions. I can picture us clustered on the second floor of a Rodeway Inn, a little group talking and laughing and looking up verses in our tiny pocket New Testaments. Nearly all those guys are out of

71

baseball now, but I wouldn't trade the hours we spent together for time in any locker room on the face of the earth.

The next year, 1982, I finally made the big jump to Triple-A baseball. I'd had an excellent year at Amarillo. My record was 15–5, with an earned run average of 2.67. All through the year, the Padres kept looking to some of the bonus babies on the team, and were disappointed that I kept topping them. But in the end they named me their minor league Player of the Year, and sent me up to Hawaii.

It was a big jump. At Double-A, you deal with dingy locker rooms and long bus trips to very unglamorous spots. Triple-A teams generally fly, and they play in big cities. Most significant of all, in Double-A you feel light-years away from the major leagues. You hope you someday make it, but it doesn't seem close. At Triple-A, many of the players have been in the majors, at least briefly.

You're only a phone call from being called up. You feel that. You feel that you're right on the verge of fulfilling all you've dreamed of.

Sadly, some of our best friends didn't make the jump to Triple-A. Byron, for example, had been injured. Within the year he was out of baseball.

But many of our Amarillo teammates moved with us. Some of them—Andy and Jackie Hawkins, Tony and Alicia Gwynn, Mark and Debbie Thurmond—would make the big leagues with us. Others—Danny and Mary Gausepohl, Jerry and Sheila DeSimone, Ron and Katie Meredith, Steve and Angie Smith—never quite got the breaks to go up and stick. But at that time we were all scrambling together, full of hope and having the time of our lives.

Tony Gwynn, by the way, started out in Amarillo with some of the worst throwing mechanics I have ever seen. His throws from the outfield were limp balloons. Never have I seen someone work as hard as he did to improve. Of course, Tony had tremendous raw ability or he would never have become the great baseball player—and outstanding outfielder—that he is today. But he wouldn't have become great without incredible work.

Janice was seven months pregnant when we moved to Hawaii. I was in Phoenix, away on a two-week June road trip, when she called. From the sound of her voice, she was in a panic. It was the middle of the night. Her water had broken. Our baby was on the way, and I was thousands of miles away. "The doctor says this is the real thing, David. I have to go in to the hospital. Can you please get here? I want you to be with me!"

The baby had been expected to arrive a few days later, just in time for a twenty-day home stand. Janice and I had been so pleased with the timing. We had congratulated ourselves on perfect planning. No one had consulted the baby.

What can you say to your wife in labor when you're thousands of miles and a big blue ocean away? I told Janice I'd get there as soon as I could, said as many encouraging words as I could think of, and hung up the phone with my head spinning. I felt excited. I couldn't believe it: our first child.

I knew Janice would be well taken care of. Many of our best friends were neighbors in the Waikiki high-rise apartment building where we had a tiny studio apartment. Half the wives were expecting first children. We all drove beat-up used cars you could hear coming. (Ours was an avocado-green Dodge Charger that had cost $750. We'd gone in with Danny and Mary Gausepohl on it, and it was the nicest car any of us had. But not nice.)

The other players' wives would be available to help Janice, even if I wasn't. But I wanted to be there. I wanted to get there as fast as I could.

I called the team's trainer, who also functioned as our traveling secretary. Waking him, I arranged to get the first plane out in the morning. Then I jumped back in bed and fell asleep. I love to sleep. And it promised to be a very long day.

I arrived in Hawaii at 11:30 Sunday morning, June 6. At 11:39, Janice gave birth to Tiffany—Tiffany, whom we'd been certain would be Joshua. I was on my way to the hospital, unfortunately, when Tiffany arrived. A couple of the wives had met me at the airport in somebody's ancient Buick station wagon, and we roared to the hospital.

I walked into the hospital about twenty minutes too late, and went right in to see Janice. When I saw her my first words were, "Hi, where's the baby?" That was definitely the wrong thing to say. Janice had been rushed to the hospital still putting curlers in her hair, because she had wanted to look nice for me. After pushing half the night, she looked awful.

Pretty soon, though, holding our baby Tiffany, we got over that bad beginning. I spent most of that day and the next at the hospital. Janice and I just couldn't believe we had gotten the most beautiful baby in the history of the world. We were really happy. Life was going amazingly well.

The following day, a Tuesday, I got up and got ready to go to the hospital again. Just as I was heading out the door, I decided to take a few more minutes to straighten up our apartment and make the bed. Janice would be coming home soon, and I wanted it to look nice for her.

The phone rang. It was Bob Cluck, the Padres' farm director. He asked about how Janice was doing. He congratulated me on Tiffany's birth.

I was a little surprised that he had called. I thought, *Hey, these people actually care.* Ballplayers sometimes have the impression that their teams consider them like a piece of meat. Yet here was an important member of the Padres' management showing appreciation for the human side of baseball.

And then he said words that roared in my brain like a jet engine. "There's actually another reason why I called. They've decided they're going to call you up. You're coming to the big leagues."

I said, "That's enough, Bob. No more jokes, okay?"

"Dave," he said, "you're coming to San Diego."

"Bob, quit messing around."

"I'm not messing around," he said. "Will you listen? We've just traded away Danny Boone. He's a left-handed reliever. We need you up here."

Only after he repeated himself three times did I understand him. Then a wave of adrenaline surged through my body. It had taken me three years to get from Double-A to Triple-A. Now, ten weeks into the season, I was getting the call. The major leagues.

I called Janice right from the apartment. I wanted her to be the first to know.

"Janice," I said, "you're not going to believe this. I just got a call from Bob Cluck."

"Oh, that's nice," she said. "Wasn't he thoughtful to call."

"Janice, listen. There's something else."

"What?" she asked.

"They're calling me up to the major leagues. We're going to San Diego."

That's when she started crying. At first I thought she was happy. Then I realized she was mad. I was bewildered. I'd called her with this wonderful news, and she was sobbing. They definitely weren't sobs of joy.

"I don't want you to go to the major leagues," she wailed. "I want you here. What am I going to do with Tiffany?"

We hadn't been together in two weeks. Janice wanted to enjoy our new baby together. Now baseball was calling me away. She was going to say good-bye, and then somehow pack our stuff, sell our car, and move, all the while caring for a baby less than a week old.

Objectively I understood what she was feeling. But I couldn't feel it with her. I was going to the majors. All my hopes of a lifetime were wrapped up in that incredibly good news.

We had a pitcher on the Triple-A team who, during spring training, had been slated for the Padres' roster. Just at the end of spring training, Dick Williams, the Padres' manager, had wanted to put him into a game. But feeling really beat, the pitcher had said he didn't want to go in. Another pitcher volunteered, and threw well. When they broke camp, he was the one selected to stay with the team. The guy who'd said no was sent down to Triple-A. In other words, I had a living reminder with me in Hawaii: You don't say no when you get the call.

I would have liked to take some time off before joining the ball club. I asked Bob Cluck whether it was possible to have a few days. But when he said they needed me immediately, I didn't complain. I said I'd be there.

I called my dad at his machine shop in Youngstown. "Hey, Dad, I was wondering if you wanted to get together for lunch," I said.

"Sure," he said, always ready to play along. "That sounds great. Where would you like to meet?"

"How about San Diego?"

"You kidding?" he said.

He was floored. I could imagine him turning cartwheels in the office. He said he'd be in San Diego pronto.

Janice and Tiffany got out of the hospital early so we could spend one day together. A sleepless night later I kissed them both good-bye.

From the San Diego airport I took a taxi directly to the clubhouse, bags and all. I didn't want to go to the hotel first. I didn't want to delay for a minute my introduction to the big leagues. I felt that a brass band should be playing as I walked in. It was, in my head.

But nobody seemed to take much notice of me.

COMEBACK

The atmosphere of the San Diego clubhouse was completely different from what I'd known in the minors. It was quiet. It was clean. Everything was neat and new. Minor league locker rooms usually have a rundown, threadbare look. There's never enough equipment. Some of the players can't even afford gloves and shoes.

Making up for it, minor league players are usually loud and enthusiastic. There's a lot of playfulness. The word for the majors is *professional.* It's as quiet as a bank in the clubhouse. You're being paid a lot of money to play the game. The clubhouse shows that seriousness.

I was thoroughly intimidated. I'm a guy who likes to play baseball as a kid's game: I yell and have fun. I couldn't behave that way around these guys. I was playing with men. They were *major league baseball players.* I wasn't sure I belonged with them. By the way they greeted me—or didn't bother to greet me—I saw they weren't sure I'd stick around. Few of them had much time for a rookie.

Doug Rader had been my manager in Hawaii. He was a little bit crazy—a player's manager who made the game fun for everybody. He yelled and hollered and got excited about the game. In San Diego, Dick Williams was a very different kind of personality. He didn't talk to his players. He certainly didn't show excitement. He had a reputation for toughness, and everything I saw indicated that the reputation was well deserved. He hardly spoke to me. I felt as though if I didn't throw well, I'd get sent back to Hawaii without a trace of human feeling.

Making It to the Big Leagues

Janice flew over with Tiffany on Saturday, six days after the birth. A lady at the airport bawled her out for traveling with such a tiny baby. The trip was long and uncomfortable. Janice could barely walk, her stitches hurt so. She spent her first ten days in San Diego in a dark Circle 8 hotel room—not the best place to spend your time with a new baby, knowing no one. My parents had come out from Youngstown, and I spent my free time traveling around town with my dad, looking for an apartment. Most wouldn't take us, because we couldn't be certain how long we'd stay. The cost of housing appalled us. We had no money until my first major league paycheck arrived.

A lot of the time I wasn't even around: I was traveling with the team. And I was pitching terribly.

It's a dreadful thing to build your life on a goal, and then sense that you're failing. I didn't have a clue on the mound. I couldn't concentrate. I felt as though the catcher was signaling me from the far side of the moon. I was lucky to get the ball to him at all, let alone hit his target. Janice could tell that something was wrong, but I wouldn't talk about it. I've always been moody; when things don't go right I keep to myself. I wasn't eating and I wasn't communicating. Janice kept saying, "What's wrong? What are you feeling?" I told her I was fine. "Are you nervous?" I said no.

I didn't know it at the time, but the Padres had called me up for a ten-day trial. If I didn't look good, they'd ship me back and call up someone else. I could feel the pressure.

COMEBACK

My low point came in San Francisco, after three weeks of poor performances. It was the Saturday Game of the Week, played under the sunlight of Candlestick Park. I saw the TV cameras and the broadcasters, and felt more intimidated than ever. The game was being broadcast all over the nation. Probably everyone who had ever known me would be watching. I was scared. I didn't want to pitch.

Yet I had to. I got the call to come in and face one left-handed batter. There were men on base, and the game was on the line. I did the worst thing a pitcher can do in that situation. I walked him.

That's not me. I'm a control pitcher. I don't walk people. But my heart was pounding and all I could hear was the crowd. Somebody was yelling, "Throw strikes!" What did he think I was trying to do?

I couldn't concentrate. I couldn't think. I could hardly see straight.

After the game Norm Sherry, the pitching coach, told me in a nice way what I knew in my heart already. "You've got to throw strikes, Dave, or they're going to send you back to Hawaii."

The next day I was up and down in the bull pen the entire game, warming up. Whether or not Dick Williams actually intended it, I believed he was keeping me up just so I could sweat bullets thinking what I had to do if I came into the game. He was tormenting me.

I was frustrated and I was scared. Mark Thurmond, one of my buddies from Triple-A ball, called me from Hawaii. He'd seen Saturday's game on TV and could tell I wasn't pitching the way I should. "Dave, don't you remember anything?" he asked me. "Are you forgetting what got you there? Be a tiger!" It was a phrase I had picked up from a Pittsburgh pitching coach. It had become practically a motto for me. "Don't nibble at those guys. Go after them!"

It was good advice, but what good would it do me? How could I tell Mark that I was just scared?

That night the team flew down to L.A., where we would face the Dodgers. Janice had driven up from San Diego with Tiffany. When the team reached the Biltmore Hotel she had already checked into my room. There she was with our baby and all the baby paraphernalia: diapers, wipes, pads, the works.

I was glad to see her, but I couldn't talk to her. The minute she saw my face she knew I was in one of my moods. "What's wrong?" she asked. She really wanted to know, and to help. But all I could say was, "I'm fine." I felt lost in my fears, cut off from humanity. I was failing. I would be sent down. I would not make it in the big leagues. All that night and the next day I acted like a caged animal. I wouldn't eat and I wouldn't talk. I was just miserable.

Early Monday afternoon, as I was preparing to leave for the game, Janice tried again. "What's wrong? I know something's wrong, David."

I think I just got tired of carrying my anxiety around by myself. I got tired of being quiet. So I told her.

I told her first what Norm Sherry had said. "I need to start throwing strikes, Janice, or they're going to send me down. Norm said that's why they brought me up, because I knew how to get the ball over the plate. But I'm not doing it."

"Well, David," she said sweetly, "why can't you throw strikes? What's wrong?"

I took a long look at her and decided I might as well say it all. "Because when I get out there I'm clueless, Janice," I said. "When I get on the mound, I don't know where I'm throwing the ball. I don't know where the plate is. I start thinking that I'm in the big leagues, and these are big league hitters, and I can't concentrate. I'm hearing everything the crowd is saying. I get the heebie jeebies. I'm scared, Janice."

For Janice it was an amazing and moving moment. She had never heard me admit to being scared. I had never opened up to her in weakness. We were talking about my feelings in a way we never had before. She began crying. She knew I couldn't cry for myself, so she cried for me.

We held each other, and talked. Mostly she talked. She said some things that made a dent in my consciousness.

"What are you afraid of?" she said. "All you can do is your best. If that's not good enough for them, so what? What's the worst thing that could happen?" She laughed. "We get sent back to Hawaii! I'd love to go. I liked it better there. I was having a blast. We'd be with all our friends again. I'd be thrilled!"

Janice has always been able to say, without fear of contradiction, that she didn't marry me for baseball. If I didn't make it in the majors, it certainly wasn't going to destroy her. I knew in many ways she'd be happy to give up the life.

If I failed, I wasn't going to lose the things that mattered. I wasn't going to lose my wife. I wasn't going to lose my daughter. I wasn't going to lose my friends.

"Are you forgetting what you've always said?" Janice asked. "Remember? You and Byron used to say you should pitch as though Jesus Christ is your only audience."

That took me back to wonderful, hot Texas days, when I'd been just a scrambling Double-A ballplayer. I'd been with some of my closest friends, playing baseball, enjoying the game, and knowing that a loving God had the only opinion of me that really mattered. Those days in Amarillo had been the happiest of my life. The reason had been, above all, that I knew who I was living for. I knew my audience.

To everybody else, you were only as good as your last performance. The pressure was relentless from the crowd, from the manager, even from the expectations of your friends and family back home. Heck, the pressure could be relentless from inside yourself. But God was concerned only that you did your best. And he was bigger than all the rest combined.

Growing up, I had always been at the center of attention. That was exactly how I had wanted it. My performance had been for me, and no one else. I had to be the star.

That kind of motivation can keep you going strong, so long as you succeed. But it's not so good for dealing with failure, or with forces beyond your control. Seeing Jesus Christ as your audience shifted the pressure off yourself. You did your best to bring glory to God, not yourself. If you lost, the loss would hurt, but it wouldn't change anything fundamental. God would still be there.

I felt better after I talked with Janice. Just letting my emotions out was a help. And her words made me remember who I was, and what really mattered.

I got into that night's game in relief. When I reached the mound I took a deep breath, looked around, and thought of Jesus as my only audience. I couldn't fail, really.

Right from the start I felt better. The batters didn't all seem like Babe Ruth. I had some rhythm to my throwing.

With two outs and Bill Russell on first, Ron Cey came up—the Penguin. Cey is proof that God didn't make baseball players in one size and shape. Ron is short and squat, and he runs with short, waddling steps. Hence the nickname.

No pitcher is wise to make fun of Cey, though. He took my pitch and roped it deep. Gene Richards went back to try to catch it, and ran face-first into the wall. Russell, going at the crack of the bat, came all the way around to score. On the throw to the plate, Cey headed for third.

The ball short-hopped Terry kennedy and bounced away. I raced after it, back to the screen. The crowd was roaring. Instead of pulling up at third, Cey saw his third-base coach waving his arm wildly toward the plate. He wanted him to score.

I caught up with the ball, pounced on it, whirled, found Terry Kennedy at the plate, and threw a strike. He put the tag on Cey, and the umpire called him out. The inning was over in a cloud of dust.

Something in me loosened up. The feeling was back. The game was fun again.

I went back to the hotel that night with a big grin on my face. Janice had been too nervous to listen to the game. But she knew as soon as she saw me that something good had happened.

"What did you do?" she asked.

I said, "I gave up a run, but I did okay. And you know what? The feeling is back."

The next night I wanted to pitch. I was anxious to get in the game for the first time since coming up to the majors.

This time I pitched three scoreless innings against the Dodgers. From that day on, I never looked over my shoulder. I pitched the way I always had. I threw strikes, and I got people out. I was in the major leagues to stay.

Janice's talk had given me more than the major leagues, however. It had planted a lesson deep in my heart. *Live life as though Jesus were your only audience.* Whenever other priorities, dreams, hopes, and fears would start to take over my mind, I'd remember that, and regain my focus.

Six years later, in Ohio, I was certainly scared while I waited for the results of my biopsy. The possibility of losing my life seemed very real. I might lose Janice, Tiffany, Jonathan. They might lose me.

But we could never lose the love of God. He was

watching over me and my family. I was conscious
of his eyes on me, his loving eyes. He was my audience. All I had to do was live for him. How could
I lose?

Diagnosis

IT had been two days since the biopsy was done on my arm—two days that had seemed like two years.

Janice has a cousin, Mark Roh, a young cancer surgeon at the M.D. Anderson Medical Center in Houston. She had called him for advice when we first heard the word "tumor." Two days after the biopsy was done, he telephoned to ask whether we had heard any results. Janice told him that we hadn't. Mark then offered to call Dr. Muschler for us.

Within an hour Mark called back. I heard Janice answer the phone in my mom's kitchen. In a moment my attention clicked in, when I realized it was he. I stood in the living room, listening to Janice's end of the conversation.

"Well, Janice," Mark said, "Dr. Muschler told me the preliminary results. It's the best it could be for what it is. If Dave had to get cancer, this is the kind you would want it to be."

"Cancer?" Janice said. I heard a note of fear in her voice. Nobody had said "cancer" before.

"Yes, that's what it is," Mark said. "It's cancer. And that's always serious. But there are many different kinds of cancer. This is the best kind of cancer to have."

He explained that my lump was a type of fibrosarcoma known as a desmoid tumor. Such a tumor was extremely unlikely to metastasize and spread through the body. It would, however, expand and spread locally. It wasn't life threatening, but it could do severe damage to my arm. The treatment called for aggressive surgery. The doctors needed to remove every last cell of the tumor.

"And I want to tell you something," Mark told Janice. "Dave needs to get it out of his body."

In our first meeting with Dr. Muschler, he'd indicated that it might be possible to watch the tumor closely and squeeze one more year out of my career. Mark spoke passionately against that option. "It's foreign," he said. "It can do nothing but harm. He needs to get it out of his body. It's cancer, and you don't mess with it."

When she hung up Janice filled in the details for me, since I'd heard only her half of the conversation. In a sense we traded emotions. For her, the word "cancer" set off alarm bells. She took on some of the worries I'd been carrying for the last two days.

For me, the overall diagnosis brought a great sigh of relief. Mark had emphasized that these were preliminary results, but I took them as final. Now I knew what I had, and I wasn't going to die of it. The doctors weren't saying "We can't be sure" any more.

I never hesitated for even a heartbeat over the operation. I wasn't going to stretch out my career at the risk of my life. Baseball had never meant that much to me.

A week later we drove up to the Cleveland Clinic to discuss the final biopsy results with Dr. Muschler. My mom came with us. She was mad: mad at God, mad at the Giants for letting the lump go untested for so long, mad over the unfairness of it all. She was just mad. Mom is a big baseball fan, and an even bigger fan of her son. She wanted to talk to the doctor herself. When we'd met with Muschler before, he'd mentioned a career threat. Mom had to hear that everything possible was being done to keep my career alive. At that point, my pitching may have meant more to her than it did to me.

Janice had a different set of concerns. She was worried about the stipulations of my contract with the Giants. She had it in her mind that since the lump had been growing before I signed, the Giants might opt out of their obligations. Or, she worried, they might insist that I try to squeeze another year out of my arm. I'd told her that the Giants weren't going to do anything like that, but I couldn't stop her worrying. When you're dealing with cancer some very irrational fears can crop up.

So we rode quietly together across the rolling farmland of eastern Ohio, each in a separate world of our own emotions. I wasn't mad or worried. I was just happy to be alive. The weather was bleak and gray, but the trees were aflame with color. We drove past the mansions of Cleveland's Shaker Heights, and near downtown pulled into the parking garage of the gleaming glass-and-steel Cleveland Clinic.

Dr. Muschler met us in an examining room, a cubicle decorated with a chart of the human skeleton. He sat behind a desk. My mom was shocked, as I had been, by how young he was. She and I were on chairs opposite him, with Janice on a seat to one side.

"The biopsy shows it's just what we suspected," Dr. Muschler said. "It's a fibrous tumor called a desmoid tumor." He spoke in a very calm and matter-of-fact manner, which I found comforting. He took out a small piece of white paper and began drawing a sketch of the deltoid muscle, showing us the location of the tumor.

"The tumor seems to be sitting right on the bone," he said. "And it's invaded the entire lower part of your deltoid, where it attaches to the bone. There are fingers going up into the main body of the muscle."

He explained again that a desmoid tumor is not life threatening. But it was a threat to my arm. Of all cancerous tumors, he said, the desmoid was probably the most likely to come back after an operation. Most cancers, when they're taken out, will return to the same site only five percent of the time or less. (They can spread to somewhere else, of course.) But studies have reported that a desmoid tumor comes back between thirty and seventy percent of the time. "If you leave one single cell in there, it can grow into another tumor. So when we do surgery, we have to do more than cut out your tumor, Dave. We have to cut it out with a wide margin all around. I'm afraid that means we'll have to take out at least half of your deltoid muscle."

He told us that the tumor was growing very slowly, and that desmoids occasionally stop growing for no apparent reason. We could, if we chose, wait and take another MRI in two or three months. If the growth stopped it might be possible to prolong my career by putting off the surgery. However, Dr. Muschler advised against that option. The tumor was close to the radial nerve, he explained, which controls sensation to the hand. If the tumor grew and damaged that nerve, I could lose use of the hand. He didn't think waiting and taking that risk was wise. Neither did I.

We began discussing the kind of surgery that was indicated. Chemotherapy or radiation, he said, would not be appropriate for this kind of tumor. As Mark had already told us, the treatment was to cut.

The problem was the humerus bone, on which the tumor was resting. "You'd normally want to take out a large margin around the tumor, just to make sure you've gotten every last cancer cell. But since it's on the bone, that's more difficult." Dr. Muschler didn't believe that the tumor had actually invaded the bone, but the most conservative approach would be to cut away half or all of the bone beneath the tumor, and reconstruct it with bone from the bone bank at the Cleveland Clinic.

He thought, though, that another option was preferable. He could cut right down to the very edge of the bone, and then freeze the portion of the tumor near the bone using liquid nitrogen. That would kill all living cells, even the living bone cells, but it would make surgery considerably less destructive and recovery much faster. With the freezing technique—cryosurgery, he called it—the bone would be brittle and liable to break for some time. But it should eventually recover its full strength.

Janice, my mom, and I took all this in rather quietly. It was a lot of information to absorb, and I can't say that I understood it all. My eyes glazed a little. What I understood was that I was going to have an operation. It would take away half my deltoid muscle. My humerus might be at risk.

My mom did not take things that easily. She began firing questions at Dr. Muschler. Couldn't he do something? Couldn't he stick a rubber band into my arm to replace the muscle? We all kind of laughed at that. It sounded ridiculous. But Dr. Muschler told us it wasn't as crazy as it sounded. He'd been talking to specialists, trying to find out whether there were such possibilities. Unfortunately, he'd found that they were more likely to inflict harm than to help.

Finally, when we'd talked through every medical angle I could think of, I asked him the question I knew was on everybody's mind—especially mine. "What about my career?" I said. I could tell he had been dancing around that subject. "Tell it to me straight, Doc. I'm not afraid."

Dr. Muschler thought for a moment and then spoke quietly. "Well, Dave, if you have this operation I think your chances of returning to professional baseball are zero."

I misunderstood him. When he said "professional" I heard "major leagues." I began talking about minor league ball. "That's okay, Dr. Muschler," I said. "I don't mind pitching minor league ball and working my way back up. Even if it takes a couple of years, that's all right." I went on talking for a minute, just thinking optimistically out loud. Janice told me later she was a little embarrassed for me. It was like I was off on a cloud, spinning dreams that had nothing to do with reality.

Dr. Muschler interrupted. "Dave, I don't think you understood me." He spoke with firm emphasis. "Losing half your deltoid muscle will take away one of the three most powerful muscles in your arm. My greatest hope is that after intensive therapy you will regain a normal range of motion and be able to play catch with your son in your backyard."

The room was very quiet.

"You mean, no professional ball at all?" I said. He said no.

There was no hesitation in my mind. "Hey, Doc, if that's the way it is, let's get on with it," I told him. "Don't think I'm going to go off in a little closet and cry. I've had a great career, I've enjoyed every minute of it, and I'm ready to go on with whatever is next."

That's what I said and what I truly felt. I told Dr. Muschler I'd been in an All-Star game. I'd pitched in two National League championships and one World Series. He was talking to a guy whom the coaches had predicted would never throw a pitch in the major leagues. I'd had a taste of every good thing baseball had to offer. What did I have to cry about?

I told him, "If I never play again, Doc, I'll know that God has someplace else he wants me. But I'll tell you something else. I believe in a God who can do miracles. If you remove half my deltoid muscle, that doesn't mean I'll never pitch again. If God wants me to pitch, it doesn't matter whether you remove all of the deltoid muscle. If God wants me to pitch, I'll be out there."

Dr. Muschler just looked at me. He must have thought I was a little crazy.

We made plans for the surgery, and I asked Muschler straight out about his qualifications. "How much of this surgery have you done?" I asked. I'd talked to Jerry Kapstein, my agent, just the day before. He'd said we would find the very best doctor in the world and go to him. I felt very comfortable with Dr. Muschler, but I wanted to be completely sure we were getting the best treatment possible. Janice and I had been praying about the decision.

To me my question was rather sensitive, but it didn't seem to bother Dr. Muschler at all. He said he'd trained at Sloan Kettering in New York, working under three doctors who had pioneered the cryosurgical procedures we would be using. While there Dr. Muschler had often used these techniques in surgery. "If I wasn't completely confident that I could do this operation as well as anyone I know of, I'd get you the doctor who could do it better."

That settled it for me. We set the date for surgery at October 7—our wedding anniversary, one year to the day after I'd won the second game of the National League championships for the Giants.

Diagnosis

* * *

It was time to tell Tiffany and Jonathan. We thought there had been enough whispered conversations out of their earshot. We shouldn't make them overhear the news. They should hear it straight from us.

As we tucked them into bed, we told them gently that I was going to need an operation on my arm, that I would be in the hospital for a while, and that I probably wouldn't be able to play baseball any more after that. We waited for the news to sink in, thinking that it would probably devastate them. We could see their minds working.

Tiffany, who was six, was first to respond. "You mean we won't have to move any more?" She was slowly thinking through the implications. "You mean I can stay in my same school? You mean we'll stay here in Ohio near Grandma and Grandpa all the time?"

Jonathan, who was three, caught on. "Dad," he said in an urgent whisper. "You mean you'll be able to play football with me every day?"

"Well, I'll have to go to work, Jonathan. But I won't be going on long trips away any more."

Spontaneously, together, Tiffany and Jonathan began to cheer.

That, as much as anything, put the operation into perspective.

Under the Knife

THE day before going in to the hospital, I made up my mind to do something I'd read in the Bible. James 5:14 says that if a person is sick he should call the elders of his church to come and pray for him. I talked to my pastor, Bob Stauffer. He wasn't sure what we could manage on such short notice, but he said he would try to round up people to meet at the church that evening.

For years Janice and I had been visiting Tabernacle Evangelical Presbyterian Church whenever we were in Youngstown. The people had offered us tremendous warmth and support, and we'd come to trust them. I especially trusted them to pray for us. Tabernacle isn't anything fancy or unusual, but its members were people who would stand by us.

When I got to the church that evening, I was surprised to find so many had come—probably close to twenty-five people. The building is colonial in style, with high ceilings and brass chandeliers. To the left of the entryway is a good-sized room where people usually gather for coffee and donuts on Sunday morning. That's where we met to pray. The men and women who had come had intensity in their eyes and in the way they shook hands. Calling the elders to pray for the sick is not something we do all the time at our church. Several other church members, hearing that the elders would be praying for me, had asked whether they could join us. They wanted to be prayed for as well.

When it came my turn, I sat in a chair in the center of the room, and the others gathered around me. Those closest put their hands on me. Bob, my pastor, had his hand on my left arm, where the operation would take place. The warmth and weight of those hands seemed to support and hold me.

Slowly, calmly, people began to pray. Their words were not what I would call "name it and claim it" prayers. They weren't trying to talk God into anything; they were just putting me firmly into his hands. They recognized his awesome power to heal, but they also recognized his desire to use people, such as doctors, to do the healing. They prayed for a peaceful and trusting attitude for me and Janice, whatever the result of the operation.

Slowly the prayers seemed to gather momentum. Seated there, surrounded by their care, I didn't have a worried bone in my body. I felt completely relaxed and at peace. I'd never felt such a thing—an awe-inspiring feeling, a sense of being lifted and held and protected by love. I didn't see how I could ever worry again.

After it was over the group slowly and quietly broke apart. There were hugs and handshakes and a few tears as we said good-bye. Bob Stauffer came up to me. "Dave," he said hesitantly, "I don't even know whether I want to tell you this. It was the weirdest thing I have ever felt. While we were praying for you, I felt my hand get extremely hot. It became so hot that I had to take it off your arm. Dave, I don't know what that means. I don't know whether that indicates some healing has taken place. But I feel very sure that God was at work tonight. We'll see the result somehow."

Bob is not the sort of person who talks wildly. He's a very sensible and down-to-earth person. I was astonished by what he said. I didn't know what it meant, but it increased my sense that a loving God was in charge of my life. As we approached the operation I didn't feel frightened at all.

The next morning Janice and I drove up to Cleveland, along with my mom. I got my blood work and half a dozen other tests done, and we spent the night at a hotel that's adjacent to the hospital. I slept well—I usually do—and checked into the hospital at 5:30 in the morning. The nurses prepped me, got me my little smock, and put me on a gurney. I kissed Mom and Janice good-bye. They seemed more worried than I was.

I felt full of high spirits as the nurses rolled me down to the operating room. I remember looking curiously at all the beeping gadgets that they'd be using during the next few hours. I told the nurses, "I just want you guys to know one thing before you put me under. A lot of people back home are praying for you right now. God's in control of this thing and I've got all the confidence in the world in every one of you. So have fun!"

One of them told me it was the first time a patient had said that people were praying for *them*. But who better to pray for? They were going to be doing the work. I was just going to be lying on my side for the rest of the day.

Dr. Muschler asked for his first instrument: a sterile marking pen. With it, he began working on my left arm, considering just where the tumor lay, and marking where he would make his incision. As he worked he explained to the two resident physicians assisting him exactly what he was doing.

I was lying on my side, propped on a bean bag to prevent pressure spots during the operation. The anesthesiologist had been with me for perhaps an hour, putting a tube into my lungs so that a machine could breathe for me, inserting IVs and a line to my arteries to measure my blood pressure, and giving me his magical cocktail of drugs. Not only was I asleep, but my muscles were paralyzed—that was why I needed the breathing machine, for my diaphragm had stopped working. My blood pressure had also been lowered to almost half normal so that I would bleed less profusely.

Using his scalpel, Dr. Muschler began to cut. Following his markings, he made an incision that started near the front of my shoulder and worked its way almost to my elbow in a long, backward-S curve. As part of the curve he made an island around the wound from my biopsy. This island—at least one centimeter wide on all sides of the original incision—he would cut away with the tumor. Since he had pulled the bit of tumor through that wound, his concern was to take away a wide margin of the skin and fat around it—anything that might have been seeded with the cancer.

Then he began to cut deeper. The wound yawned open naturally, like a mouth opening into my arm. His cutting stopped short of the tumor itself. The tumor was enclosed within the sac of fibrous tissue that surrounds the deltoid muscle, the fascia. He did not want to break it. During the operation, he would always keep a margin of flesh between his scalpel and the tumor itself. He wanted not to see the tumor, even when he peeled it off the bone.

So he went around the tumor. It was located on the narrowing triangle of muscle where the deltoid dives between the triceps and biceps muscles. Dr. Muschler found the biceps—this is the muscle that boys flex when they are "showing off their muscle"—and with a long incision cut open its fascia. The fascia is a tough, white membrane enclosing each muscle.

With his fingers inside the biceps muscle compartment, he pushed the biceps muscle away from the tumor, working his way through the muscle fibers clear to the humerus bone. He inserted metal retractors against the bone to hold the muscle back.

He did the same thing on the other side of the tumor, going through the triceps muscle compartment. On both sides, he snipped carefully so that he left some normal muscle against the fascia that contained the tumor.

As he approached the bone he carefully identified the radial nerve, which followed the humerus. If this nerve were damaged my hand could become a claw. Dr. Muschler protected the nerve with sponges beneath his metal retractor.

He could now see to the bone, exposed on both sides of the tumor. Dr. Muschler was prepared to make the cut that would make all the difference. Having separated the deltoid muscle compartment from its neighbors, he was ready to cut the deltoid in two.

He measured carefully again, making sure that he took off four centimeters of healthy muscle above the tumor. And then he cut. The line ran at about the halfway point on the muscle. A sense of the pity of it struck Dr. Muschler. It was the largest deltoid muscle he had ever seen: healthy, vibrant, strong, a heavy mass of meat. He was quite sure that he was cutting away my career.

It has been widely reported that Dr. Muschler took away half my deltoid muscle. That, while correct, understates what he did. A muscle must be attached at both ends. Otherwise it is as useless as a broken rubber band. Dr. Muschler had essentially made the remaining deltoid muscle like a broken rubber band. A few connecting tissues tied it to the bone above where he had cut. But the far greater proportion of connective tissue had been severed. Half the muscle was gone, but at least ninety-five percent of its function was destroyed. Essentially, I would have to learn to live without a deltoid muscle.

Then came the last and most difficult part of the surgery: separating the tumor from the bone.

There is a tough, thick sheath on every human bone, a living tissue called the periosteum. Taking an electrocautery scalpel, Dr. Muschler burned through this sheath on the humerus, incising a line on both sides of the bone at least five millimeters (about a quarter inch) from the tumor, then cutting across the bone above and below where the deltoid attached. He had made a rough ellipse on the periosteum, an ellipse that enclosed the tumor. Cryosurgery would kill every living cell within this area before he removed it from the bone.

He had a little hand spray gun, something like a power paint spray gun, but filled not with paint but with liquid nitrogen. He and his assistants began spraying a one centimeter strip near the line he had cut on the bone. Frost quickly developed on the tissue. They waited until it thawed thoroughly—that took fifteen minutes—then sprayed again. After a second thawing, it was frozen a third time, then thawed a third and final time. Dr. Muschler took up a blunt instrument called an elevator, which looks like a broad-headed screwdriver. With it he pried up the edge of now-dead tissue on my bone, staying a quarter inch away from any tissue which had not yet been frozen. He said it was a little like prying a thick layer of paraffin off a tin can. Immediately the freezing began again, spraying another one centimeter wedge of tissue, thawing it, freezing and thawing it again, freezing and thawing it a third time. This triple cycle was done approximately ten times before the last of the tumor could be pried free from the bone.

And then the tumor, all of it, surrounded by a layer of muscle and fat and fascia and frozen periosteum, could come out whole. Dr. Muschler lifted it gently out of my arm and handed it to one of his assistants. Surgeons have a special, ironic term for this. They say they "harvest" a tumor. After the harvest, Dr. Muschler cleaned the wound and prepared to close me up.

I did not see any of this, of course; I only heard about it later. I wish I could have seen it. I wish that I had asked Dr. Muschler to keep the tumor for me in a jar, so I could have seen the alien that was cut out of my body.

Janice and my mom sat in a large, modern waiting room, filled with people whose loved ones were apparently in for far more serious operations than I. Some were waiting for news of life and death. They waited quietly, tensely, anxiously.

The room had a large front desk. Periodically the receptionist would call out a name, the family would go to the desk, and she would tell them whatever news had reached her. Usually, she would say that the patient was out of surgery and in recovery; the surgeon would be down in a minute to talk. There was a small, private conference room for the family and their doctor.

All morning Janice and my mom watched the constant flow of people and doctors, and heard no news of me. I had been wheeled away well before 7:00, and Dr. Muschler had predicted that the operation would take four hours. By noon they began to feel slightly anxious.

Janice had hoped and prayed that the doctors would cut open my arm and find nothing. The cancer would have disappeared, or turned into mere scar tissue. As the hours passed, that hope faded.

Fears about the unknown entered in. Janice found a pay phone and began calling friends, collect. She needed support; she needed someone to talk with.

It was not until 1:30 in the afternoon that Janice was called to the receptionist's desk. Dr. Bergfeld, who was observing Dr. Muschler at work, was on the line from the operating room.

"It's a lot more involved than we had expected," he said. "They're just doing the cryosurgery now. It's going fine, everything is going to be all okay. He's going to be handicapped all right, but don't worry." His powerful voice was comforting, even if it evaporated whatever hope of a miracle Janice had remaining. "I don't want you to worry," he said. "We're going to get this boy back in shape. We feel like we've gotten all of the tumor." He kept referring to what marvelous hands Dr. Muschler had.

Janice's mind was full of scattered thoughts: a fleeting disappointment that the tumor had not disappeared, worry over the handicap Dr. Bergfeld had mentioned, anxiety that perhaps he was not telling everything. The day had begun to seem cruelly long. She was praying constantly.

Hours more passed without a word. The afternoon began to grow dark, and the population of the waiting room dwindled. My mom became quieter as the day wore on. Dad had arrived from work, and he sat with them. He, too, who usually talks a blue streak, was quiet.

Janice went to a pay phone and for the second time called Jenny Hammaker. She and Jenny are as close as Atlee and I. With her, Janice could let down and release her fears. When she heard

Jenny's voice, tears came into her eyes. She asked Jenny to keep praying. She didn't understand why it was taking so long.

At about 3:30 in the afternoon one of my mom's cousins walked in. Jerry works at the Cleveland Clinic, but had no idea that I was being operated on. "Donna, what are you doing here?"

My mom is not a crier; she normally holds her emotions in very tightly. But she completely lost control. She began sobbing and crying hysterically. "He's been in there too long, we don't know what they're doing with him. They're maiming my son, Jerry, they're maiming him!"

Jerry held her and tried to calm her. The emotions played themselves out, and my mom settled down to wait again. The last families were called to the receptionist's desk, were met by their doctors, talked privately and left. Finally at 5:15, nearly eleven hours after I had been wheeled in, the receptionist told Janice that I was in recovery. The doctor would be coming to meet her in a moment.

But he didn't come. Surprise turned to irritation turned to concern turned to fear. Three-quarters of an hour passed, and still Dr. Muschler didn't arrive.

The Aftermath

I awoke in the recovery room feeling awful. I could hear, but I couldn't get my eyes open. The drugs remaining in my body made me feel horrible. And I was in excruciating pain, worse pain than I had ever felt in my life. It did not come from my arm. It came from somewhere in the lower part of my body.

I can handle plenty of pain. Most of the time people have no idea I'm even feeling it. But I had no way to hide this pain, and no desire. I moaned and I cried.

I remember hearing the doctors' voices, and feeling their hands, even though I couldn't keep my eyes open, or focus on anything when I did. My mind was not working clearly.

I remember thinking, *What is this pain?* The doctors were asking the same question. They began poking me and asking, "Is that it? Does that hurt?" It hurt everywhere they touched me. Finally they poked a spot on my leg, and I felt as though I jumped high enough to touch the ceiling. "You got it that time, Doc."

I heard them talking, though I had no idea what they said. They asked me questions that I must have answered, though I don't remember how. Nurses were scurrying after instruments. I gathered that my problem was something unusual. All I really remember was the pain. Finally Dr. Muschler leaned over me and told me that they would have to take me back into the operating room for an emergency fasciotomy.

I said, "That's okay, Doc, just do what you have to do. Just relieve the pain. Put me to sleep so I don't have to feel it any more."

Dr. Muschler finally arrived in the waiting room at six o'clock. Janice's heart went out to him, he looked so exhausted and sad. His complexion was gray, and he was drenched in sweat. He's a tall, slender man, and he drooped like a wilted flower. He struggled for words. "I don't even want to tell you this," he said. "The surgery was so beautiful, I really should be ecstatic right now, but I have to take him back in for emergency surgery on his leg."

He explained briefly what had happened. Apparently my thighs are so muscular that they bulge out more than a normal individual's. With my blood pressure reduced by the anesthesia during the long operation, the pressure of lying on my side had cut off the flow of blood to my thigh muscle. After the operation, when my blood pressure was increased, the blood-starved muscle had swelled massively and cut off the supply of blood again. It's an unusual injury known as compartment syndrome; it's most often seen in people who have been crushed in an accident. The classic symptom of compartment syndrome is blinding pain. If allowed to continue for too long, compartment syndrome can cause the muscle tissue to die.

Dealing with it was simple. They had to cut into my leg and cut open the fascia. With the muscle compartment open, the pressure on my leg would be relieved and blood flow restored.

For two more hours Janice and my mom sat in the waiting room. The playoffs between the Dodgers and the Mets were on TV, and they half-watched that. My dad had had to leave for home. All the other familes were gone; the room was empty except for them. Finally the receptionist told them that Dr. Muschler was on his way.

Hope does not die easily, and Janice was still clinging to the very faint possibility that he might say everything had turned out okay, that the cancer had disappeared, that a miracle had happened. He didn't. He sat down with her and told her that my leg was fine, that the operation on my arm had gone very well, but that they had needed to take fifty percent of my deltoid muscle as he had expected. He said that this would drastically affect certain kinds of movement. For example, I might never be able to reach into my back pocket with my left arm to extract my wallet. He hoped I would be able to lift my arm over my head again, but it would not be easy. I would need plenty of therapy to regain that kind of motion.

"In other words," Janice said after she'd asked all the questions she could think of. "In other words, short of a miracle, he'll never pitch again."

Janice's memory of this moment is crystal clear. Dr. Muschler, still wearing his blue surgical gown, looked her in the eye and repeated the words back. "That's right," he said. "Short of a miracle, he will never pitch again."

When I woke up in recovery again, I was in excruciating pain. Janice and my mom came in, and when I saw the reaction on their faces I knew that I looked truly terrible. My arm and my leg were wrapped in huge bandages; I had gauges and tubes all over me. And I was moaning from pain and thirst.

As I was all drugged up, I can't remember anything very clearly, but I do remember a very pretty nurse who would not let me drink any water. Finally when Dr. Muschler said I was all right, she relented and let Janice get a popsicle out of the freezer for me. The first one, I remember, was red. Janice fed it to me, leaning over me and tenderly putting the red ice to my lips. I sucked it down like a man who's been lost in the desert for a week. After I had gone through all the popsicles Janice fed me ice from a cup. I was insatiably thirsty. Janice and my mom were allowed to stay with me in recovery for some time. I spent the night there, a difficult, drugged night of pain.

The next morning I felt worse, if anything. I had a desperate feeling that I had to get out of that recovery room with all its noise and commotion. Nobody else seemed in any hurry to see me move, though. They kept coming for other people, and passing me by. Finally a guy came for me, and I was rolled down to my room. I had a roommate, though it would be a while before he registered with me. I was in too much pain. He told me later,

"Man, when you came in I thought you were going to die. You were in bad, bad shape."

Being under anesthesia for so long had knocked my body systems out of whack; they felt as though they were running in reverse. My arm was numb. They had partly frozen the ulnar nerve, which runs along the humerus bone, so my hand was weak and some feeling was gone. For days I felt a buzzing in my arm, like you get when you bump your funny bone.

My leg, however, was fully awake and screaming for mercy. I had a morphine pump, and I could give myself a shot any time. The only trouble was, when I'd used up my dosage there wasn't any more in the pump, so I was pumping nothing. That didn't keep me from exercising that pump constantly.

I told Janice that I had to call Atlee. She told me I was crazy, but I insisted. She dialed the number and got Atlee on the line. I tried to talk to him, but it was too hard even to hold on to the receiver. Atlee kept saying, "Are you all right?" He could understand only every third or fourth word. I finally dropped the receiver. Janice picked it up and told Atlee I was in no shape to talk.

When you feel that bad you can't live. You just survive. Somehow I got through the day. The aftereffects of the drugs wore off, and my body began to feel like it belonged to me again. My pain was still bad, but the possibility of living began to seem attractive.

My roommate, a guy named Al, was a delight. He hadn't wanted to say anything the first day I'd come in, because he wasn't sure if I would make it through the night. After I began perking up, we had a lot of fun together. We had a gorgeous black nurse who looked like Clair Huxtable on "The Cosby Show." She would get us midnight snacks, sit and talk to us, and generally treat us like royalty. We watched the Mets go down to the Dodgers in the playoffs.

On the second day of recovery they took my urinary catheter out. After a while I had to pee, bad. Janice and my mom were there. I told them there was no way I could go in the bedpan.

They said, "Just lie there and go to the bathroom."

I said, "You're crazy, I'm not going to do that."

Until that point I had not been able to get out of bed, or even think about it. The doctors want you to get up and around as soon as possible, though. They had ordered up a wheelchair for me, and a male nurse helped me get out of bed and into it. Janice was going to wheel me around the hospital. My mom had gone.

"Janice," I said after the nurse had gone, "wheel me over to the bathroom." The feeling was growing more and more urgent.

"No, I'm not going to," she said. "You're in no shape. You're supposed to use the bedpan."

I said, in my most menacing strong male voice, "Get me over there now."

"No," she said. She was ready to fight me on it, I could tell. She thought if I got in there I might pass out, or rupture my stitches.

"Janice!"

She finally gave in, wheeled me over to the door

and helped me to my feet. She was going to assist me inside.

As soon as I got up and in the door, I shut it on her and locked it. Hospital bathrooms are terrific, with railings everywhere, and with my one functioning leg and one functioning arm I could manage pretty well. Janice was screaming, "Get the nurse! Get the nurse!"

"Stay out of here! I'm all right!"

The nurse came. He couldn't believe it. "Oh my goodness," he was saying, "do you know the kind of trouble I'm going to get into? Let me in."

"Leave me alone!" I yelled back. "I'm all right!"

But I wasn't. Balancing there on one leg, I couldn't go. My body simply would not operate. I was so angry I wanted to spit fire. Finally I had to give up, open the door, and get back in my wheelchair.

For at least another hour I endured. Janice left to go back home. My brother Joey came with his wife Gina. We were visiting, sort of, but it was difficult to talk feeling the way I did. Finally I asked the two of them to take a hike. Gina left while Joey helped me get out of bed. He hung around until I told him I didn't need an audience. Would he go walk around with his wife? After about ten minutes balanced on one leg, my head leaning against the wall, I was able to do what I needed to do. I filled an entire cup, a big one. It was the best feeling I'd had in weeks. I was so proud of myself I called Janice to share the news.

The next day I got wheeled to the therapist for the first time. He got me on the stationary bike to see if I could get some mobility back in my leg. I was able to bend my knee a little. My arm I couldn't move at all, so he held it and took it through a range of motion for me. The idea was to simply get the muscles and joints moving again. Otherwise I might be left with permanent stiffness, or have to fight harder to regain motion later.

After five days in the hospital they released me. It was a bitterly cold, gray day, with flurries of snow blowing across the road. The air felt wonderful to me. I'd almost forgotten there was an outdoors.

Getting me out of the wheelchair and in the car door was a monumental process. I couldn't grab anything with my left arm, which was in a sling, or push off with my right leg. I had a cane for walking, which I set beside me on the seat. I finally made it in. Then I told Janice where to go. "Take me to Arby's!"

The Arby's chain originated in Youngstown. Janice and I have been eating at Arby's since we were high school honeys. During college, when she had a job, I used to get her to pay—and then I'd use my money to take out other girls. I don't know why she ever forgave me.

My appetite had returned, and as my family and my teammates can tell you, it is a healthy appetite. I hadn't had a decent meal since I had gone into the hospital. I munched down my standard Arby's order—one hot ham-and-cheese sandwich, one turkey deluxe, with curly fries—and felt much better.

On the way home we stopped at our new house. I wanted to see what the contractor had done since

I'd left for the hospital. For Janice, watching me hobble around with my cane, my eyes half shut from the beginning of a blinding headache, it was a very sad moment. She saw a man who had been strong and vital a week before. Now he looked pitiful. He couldn't even walk without help.

We drove on to my parents' house. Jonathan and Tiffany had not come up to the hospital during my stay, so they were ready to hug in a big way. Unfortunately, there really wasn't any part of my body they could hug without half killing me. But it was wonderful to see them.

Mom was cooking dinner. The operation was over. I had made it through one set of obstacles. A whole obstacle course—many, many more barriers—lay ahead.

In the Dungeon

I came home to live in my parents' basement—
what Janice and I called the dungeon. There at the
bottom of steep stairs, in the darkness next to the
family pool table, in front of an old unused wet bar,
and nearly buried under various boxes and papers, was—and is—one of the most brutally uncomfortable foldout couches in America. We slept
on its lumps and ridges for slightly over a month,
until our house was completed.

I should say we *tried* to sleep. Normally, I am
a thrasher. I destroy my bed every night. Now I
had to lie flat on my back. If I rolled to one side
or the other the pain was unbearable. Sleeping flat
on my back meant that I didn't sleep. I dozed fit-
fully. I lay awake squirming, wondering whether
a comfortable position existed. The pain from my
leg would gradually increase, and I grew more and
more wretched as my pain medicine wore off.
With one functioning arm and one functioning leg
I would try to inch my way up into a sitting position. Janice would hear me, would awaken. I
would feel her getting up, then hear her running
water in the bathroom upstairs. She came back

down the stairs with a glass of water and two more pain pills for me. I would fall into a doped-up haze.

To add to it, Jonathan never slept through the night. We would hear him crying upstairs, and Jan would stumble up to get him. I would have helped, but it was extremely difficult for me to even get off the bed using only one arm and one leg, let alone to climb those steep stairs with my cane.

Then there was the midnight monster. Some sort of animal had taken up residence in the ceiling overhead, and while we lay awake we would hear him skittering above us. Once he fell through, right onto the bed, and woke us up bolt upright before disappearing into the darkness.

So neither Janice nor I slept much. I tried every position. I tried sleeping upstairs on the couch. Nothing worked. I eventually gave up trying, and decided I would have to live on four hours of semi-sleep a night.

That Thursday night I watched the Dodgers play the fifth and final game of the World Series, finishing off the A's. It wasn't a very close game. With Orel Hershiser on the mound, it was obvious the A's hitters were overmastered.

Janice went to bed, but I remained upstairs. The sofa felt as comfortable as my bed in the basement, so I thought I might as well stay put. The room was dark except for the dim light from the TV.

I never cry. I would like to be able to shed tears, to express my feelings more freely, but I am not someone who can.

I saw Orel make the last pitch of the game, striking out Tony Phillips. I saw him throw a quick glance to heaven, thanking God. I saw him engulfed in the surging, pulsating mass of Dodger blue.

I had been rooting for the National League. I was truly happy for Orel, knowing that he shares my faith in Christ and that he is an admirable human being. Yet I couldn't help thinking how the season had begun for me against the Dodgers. I had been the dominant pitcher. It had looked like my year. It could have been me on that mound.

Instead, it appeared that I was done with baseball.

So I cried. All alone, lit only by the flickering TV, I broke into big, fat tears.

Every day that week I got a cluster headache. Only they could make me forget the pain in my leg, because they hurt one hundred times worse.

I'd first gotten them in college. They'd come at the same time each day, while I was driving to my English Composition class. Maybe that was the cause. Suddenly, boom, I had a headache just over my eyes that I thought would kill me.

I'd had them again in Colombia, when I was playing winter ball. I remember sitting outside our bedroom with a pillow behind my head, slamming my head repeatedly against the wall.

And now they were coming again, every day like clockwork. I got a headache one day while Janice was driving that turned me completely insane. I was screaming at her to drive faster, and pounding my foot on the floor like I could break a hole in the steel. Doctors have told me that people with cluster headaches sometimes put their heads through walls in an effort to stop the pain. That's not hard for me to imagine. When I had one, Janice and the kids could only leave the room. They couldn't help me, and I was not pleasant company.

I love my parents very much, but sharing their house was hard. They naturally wanted to be part of our life, and we naturally wanted to be by ourselves. Janice and I had financial decisions to make. We had to think about a career outside of baseball. My parents were intent on thinking positively, and became very upset when Janice or I would discuss the medical realities as the doctors had told them to us.

The Giants called up and wanted to know our plans for spring training. Spring training! That seemed as likely as a trip to the moon.

Every day we drove over to check what the workmen were doing on our house. I would walk slowly through the rooms, hobbling with my cane, trying to imagine what life would be like there. The work seemed to go very slowly.

And yet, as gloomy as this sounds, as gloomy as it really was, it contained the light of genuine hope. We discovered that our faith was real.

You always wonder how it will be to go through a difficult time. You talk about the love of God, yet you can't help wondering: When tough times come will you really be able to live it? We found that we could. We found that faith carried us through our troubles, day by day.

The first Sunday after getting out of the hospital we went to church. We purposely arrived a bit late, so I would not have to greet too many people as I hobbled painfully in. We found a seat in the very back. People sneaked a peek at me and quickly looked away. I was a painful sight, limping slowly with a cane, my arm in a sling. My face told the story of the battle I was in.

In our church we sometimes have a time when anybody can stand up and share what's happening to them—either thanking God, or asking for prayer. I hadn't planned on participating, but when others began sharing, I made up my mind I had something to say. I rose slowly to my feet, balancing with my cane.

"I want to praise God," I said, "for your prayers." I spoke very slowly, because as soon as I got up, my emotions ran away from me. "I want you to know how much it meant, that people here were praying for me." My voice began cracking. I was struggling for control, and then suddenly crying. That made the second time in the week, and this time in public. "During the whole week at the hospital," I said, "I had a tremendous sense of peace. I felt the presence of God with me. I knew that my faith and your prayers made a difference."

Janice, sitting next to me, was falling apart. I was dripping a few tears; she was a fountain. She had seen me cry exactly once before that, many years ago when she'd broken our engagement and I'd known that only tears would make her change her mind. I'd often kidded her how hard I'd worked to make those tears come.

Now I was crying in church. They were tears of thankfulness, not grief. "I've come to the place," I said, "where if I never play baseball again it's okay with me."

*   *   *

Scott and Kathy Garrelts, two of our best friends on the Giants, came to visit. They were driving through the area, and stopped to spend a quiet day with us. Scott isn't a talkative guy anyway, and the sight of me dragging around like an invalid shook him. He kept taking long, silent looks at me.

He went with me to therapy. I'd been very fortunate to find Ken Johnson, a physical therapist who had worked with Dr. Bergfeld at the Cleveland Clinic, practicing nearby. Scott stood by and watched as Ken took my arm through a series of exercises. He had to do it all for me, as though he were working with a big, floppy mannequin. Driving back Scott didn't say much. Later he told Atlee Hammaker that I just wasn't the same old Dave.

I talked to Atlee fairly often. We talked baseball, discussing whatever news was in the paper about trades and free agents. But when it came to discussing our personal lives, I didn't have much to say. I remember one lusterless November day when Atlee asked me what I was doing. All I could think was that I'd spent hours by the window, watching some construction going on across the street. That was it. Atlee couldn't believe he was talking to Dave Dravecky.

I got some encouragement when I had my stitches checked at the Cleveland Clinic two weeks after the surgery. I mentioned the headaches, and they sent me to see a neurologist who immediately diagnosed them and gave me a powerful drug to knock them out.

The fun part, though, was seeing Dr. Muschler.

In the Dungeon

Before he came in, one of his young residents checked me out. He asked me to try to lift my arms. I was able, with some effort, to take them up over my head. The surprise registered all over his face. "Wait until Muschler sees this," he said.

When Dr. Muschler came in I didn't let on what I could do. I just waited until he asked me to lift my arms. Then I slowly lifted them straight over my head. I wasn't disappointed by his reaction. "That's amazing," he said.

But when he had me try other motions, it was more discouraging. The worst was a very simple one: with my hands at my sides, I tried to move my left arm straight back. Pushing and straining, I couldn't move it more than two inches.

Without a functioning deltoid muscle, I had lost certain kinds of motion. The purpose of therapy was to retain my shoulder to use other muscles. But there was no guarantee that the full range of motion would return. A lot of it depended on my motivation.

I worked hard. One day about three weeks after getting my stitches checked, I came home from my therapy workout and found Janice washing the dishes. My mom's kitchen is stepped up a bit above a breakfast nook which overlooks their backyard. I walked in from the driveway and stood looking up at Janice.

"Hey, I've got something to show you," I said.

"Yeah?" she said.

"Yeah. Watch this."

Using my left arm, I slowly reached behind me to my rear pants pocket. I took out my wallet and set it down on the counter, where I always put it when I came home.

Janice was making little leaps of joy, her hands clasped in front of her. "Oh, wow," she said. It was the move Dr. Muschler had said would take months of rehabilitation to regain.

"That's not all," I said. "Watch this."

I stepped up into the kitchen area, where she could see me clearly, and stood for a moment cradling an imaginary baseball in my hand. Then slowly and deliberately, I went through my pitching motion. Plant your foot, lift your hands to your chest, pivot, lift your hand behind your ear, throw. My motion felt the way it always had—slower and sorer, but essentially the same.

Janice just stared. Tears began popping into her eyes. We hugged each other. "I can't believe it," she said.

That was the day we really began to hope I would pitch again.

Comeback?

ON November 18, six weeks to the day after my operation, we moved into our new home. It was a lovely, warm day, almost balmy for November. Tiffany and Jonathan were fascinated by the moving truck. They spent most of their morning marching in and out of it. I limped happily around the house with my cane, enjoying looking at furniture I hadn't seen since we left San Diego in July.

After weeks in the dungeon, our new house felt as big as a gymnasium. It's a two-story brick home with lots of light and an open, airy feel. It gave me a wonderful sense of space.

While we were moving in the plumbers were finishing their work. All of a sudden we heard water dripping, and then saw a cascade of water dropping from the kitchen ceiling, out of the smoke alarm. Soon waterfalls were plummeting down all over the house. The plumbers were running up and down, shouting. But Janice and I couldn't stop laughing. It was a big joke.

Somebody said they couldn't believe we were laughing.

"Why not?" Janice said. "Some day ten years

from now we'll all sit back and laugh at this. We might as well start now."

Our house seemed too beautiful to spoil with something minuscule like plumbing. We were so, so happy to finally live in our own home. It felt like a new beginning. Comeback? Just a few weeks before the idea had seemed ridiculous. The doctors had told us to forget it, and anybody who looked at me after the operation would have agreed. When the Giants called asking about my plans for spring training, Jan had been annoyed. "Why can't they just leave him alone?"

But after I'd shown Janice the wallet move and the pitching motion, possibilities and hopes had seemed to spring up like May daffodils. We quickly began playing the "What if . . ." game.

Realistically, though, we were getting ahead of ourselves. I had removed my wallet from my back pocket. That was somewhat different from pitching major league baseball.

When I'd started therapy, Dr. Muschler had warned us not to look for the light at the end of the tunnel. "Don't look at whether or not you'll play baseball," he'd said. "Focus on getting back normal use in your arm. When you get normal use, then focus on rebuilding arm strength. After the strength comes back, start looking at developing the muscles to throw a baseball. Then, if that happens, start focusing on throwing the ball. Just take it in sequence. Don't look ahead to try and see everything. Focus on each day."

I suspect most people, if they haven't done it, think that rehabilitation therapy is no big deal. I found it mentally and physically draining. It was demanding work, and yet often seemed piddly and pointless. We started with Ken simply holding my arm and taking it through a range of motions. Then I got to Velcro a one-pound weight on my wrist. For an hour I moved that tiny one-pound weight around. What's more, at the end of the hour I felt exhausted.

Very slowly I moved from one-pound weights to two-pound weights, then to three-, four-, and eventually five-pound weights. I tried to put the end result out of my mind. I couldn't know where it would lead. All I knew was that I had work to do. I was willing to put forth every ounce of energy and exhaust every avenue to regain as much use of my arm as possible.

I'm a professional athlete. By definition that means I've not only tried to be in control of my destiny, I have generally succeeded. Nobody else thought I would make it to the major leagues, but I took my destiny in my own hands—at least, so I thought—and made it.

But with cancer there were huge ranges of concern that I couldn't control. I couldn't just think positively and visualize success and make the arm behave as though there was a whole deltoid muscle. I wanted to come back and play again, but wanting it wouldn't make it so.

Sometimes, for long periods, I seemed to make no progress at all. Janice would have to talk to me to get me going. She sometimes had to push me out the door to my therapy sessions. I always felt much better when I came home after a workout, though, knowing I'd done what I could.

I was enough of a realist to know that the odds

were against my coming back. I knew I might not make it. My part, I believed, was to do everything possible, to try with all my might. Then, if I couldn't pitch, God would have other, better things for me to do. My faith in a personal God released me from the fear of failing. That's not fatalism. It's trust. Trust helped me to work hard and not to worry about the outcome.

Perhaps I ought to mention that I was working in obscurity. Of course, Youngstown people knew about me and were always interested, but I didn't hear much from out-of-town reporters during the winter. Most of them, hearing I'd been operated on for cancer in my pitching arm, probably felt sorry for me but mentally crossed me off their list. There was one exception. A reporter for the *San Jose Mercury News,* Tim Cowlishaw, flew out just before Christmas and spent the day with me. He went to therapy and watched my workout. We talked for several hours.

Janice and I were quite surprised that he'd come from so far away. We were even more surprised when we saw the story. It had been plastered across the front of the sports page on Christmas Day, and took up four columns inside the sports section as well. The headline read, "All he needs is a miracle." What amazed us most was how extensively the story talked about my faith in Jesus Christ. Previously, reporters hadn't considered it newsworthy. Somehow, when cancer came into the picture, faith was news.

*　　　*　　　*

Comeback?

By Christmas I was pretty psyched up about my recovery. My leg was feeling fine. I had recovered a full range of motion in my arm, though it was still very weak. On January 9, a Monday, I was scheduled to meet with the doctors at the Cleveland Clinic. I knew I was going to surprise them. I relished the thought of amazing them. That's a residue from my days as an underdog.

Janice and I drove up to the Cleveland Clinic with Ken Johnson, my therapist. We were all excited, yet we felt tremendous uncertainty. We had invested a great deal in my recovery. So had the doctors we were about to meet. We—Janice, Ken, and I—knew some things about my body's response that the doctors didn't and the doctors knew some medical facts that we didn't. The two half-orbs were about to join.

We walked quickly through the modern, airy, glass-and-steel halls of the clinic. Soon we were in a tiny examining room, waiting for the doctors. Dr. Bergfeld's entourage came in first: young residents in their white coats and ties, all excited and full of good cheer.

Janice felt like a little mouse, just watching from the corner to see what would happen. Every time I'd made progress, she'd cheered me on, but she could never let herself get too optimistic. When she'd looked ahead, she'd seen far too many obstacles. Yet she had caught the excitement I was feeling.

"Okay, Dave," one of the doctors said, "go through the motions for us. Show us what you can do."

I did it like a showman. First I performed the

movements I knew wouldn't surprise them, like reaching over my head. Then I worked into the motions that I knew would blow them away, like starting with my hand at my side and pushing it straight back, or starting with my hand at my side and lifting it straight out from my body.

I got the response I was looking for. "Wow, Dave, that's good. That's pretty impressive."

But the fun really began after they filed out and Dr. Muschler came in. He was friendly and kind, and as before I got a wonderful sense of security from him. After the bare minimum of small talk he examined my arm and then asked me to go ahead and show him what I could do. He didn't say anything until I got to the point of pushing my arm back from a position at my side. I could go as far back with my left arm as with my right.

Muschler said, "How are you doing that?" He came up to me and put his hands on my shoulder. "Do it, Dave." So I did it. "Do it again." He was feeling my muscles work, trying to understand what was moving my arm. In a low, thinking-to-himself voice, he said, "You must be using your lats." Then he stepped back and stared at me, as though he were looking for a trick. He went over to a chair in the corner of the room and from then on just sat there, not talking unless someone asked him a question.

Dr. Bergfeld came in, with his complete entourage. There were five doctors in that tiny room, plus the three of us. Dr. Bergfeld's exuberant presence seemed to take up the space of two or three extra people.

"Well, Dave, how are you doing?" he asked. I

said I was doing great, and began going through the motions for him. He started crowing. "You see?" he said to Muschler. "You see? I told you that you weren't dealing with an ordinary individual here. He's an athlete, and they're different."

Dr. Muschler just sat in his corner, saying, "I'm really impressed."

"Hey, Doc," I said, "it's just because of the terrific job you did in there. Thanks a lot."

We were all talking at once and celebrating together. Then came a pause. Bergfeld looked at Muschler. "Well," he boomed, "let's get him throwing! What do you think, George? Can he throw?"

Throw? All these months I had not so much as picked up a baseball. Never once had I cradled that little white orb in my hand and felt its solid, smooth weight. Dr. Muschler had warned me against throwing anything. I hadn't picked up a rock and thrown it against a tree, I hadn't tossed a piece of paper into the wastebasket. I'd done my workouts with my little wrist weights. Throw? Throw!

Janice, listening to the last of the obstacles come down, almost burst with excitement.

Muschler, however, was quite cautious. The humerus bone, he said, was very brittle because of the freezing he'd done to kill the cancer cells. A sizable portion of the bone had died and was in the process of repairing itself.

All the x-rays indicated that healing was going well. But we were moving into an area of the unknown. Muschler said that when whole bones were frozen, they were prone to fracture for a year or two after surgery. Mine, though, should recover more quickly, since they had only frozen one surface of the bone.

But Muschler was concerned that if we went too quickly, the area of dead bone might crack before the rest of the bone had grown strong enough to take over. The whole bone might snap. Muschler felt that we would need to work very carefully, gradually increasing the level of my activity. Even then, we would be taking a risk. There was no track record to follow. No one had ever tried to throw baseballs ninety miles an hour after having his bone frozen, much less tried it without a deltoid muscle.

Dr. Muschler didn't feel that I could throw all out before April. He thought we had to allow a full six months for healing.

"So no spring training?" Dr. Bergfeld said. "You don't think he could go down there and take light workouts?"

Muschler thought if I got down to spring training, with all my teammates, there would be a temptation to say, "Forget those doctors," and let it rip. He was right, too.

Bergfeld was funny, though. He understands athletes, and he knew what spring training was really all about. He laughed and said, "Come on, doctor, this boy needs a vacation! We've got to recommend to the Giants that he go to spring training so that he can get a little vacation in. Maybe we should recommend he go to the Bahamas or something. The boy has been working hard."

"Well, maybe he can go for the last week,"

Muschler said. "But I don't want him to interrupt his therapy."

I just watched and listened as these two great doctors went back and forth over my treatment. Whatever they came up with, I was charged up. For the first time the doctors were talking as though baseball was a possibility.

They finally decided that they would let me start throwing a football. They explained that because of the football's weight, I couldn't develop nearly the arm speed that I would with a baseball. A slower speed would protect my bone from the tremendous torque developed when a ball is released. Also, a football is less forgiving in terms of the proper mechanics of throwing. There are a million and one ways to throw a baseball, most of them wrong, but if you're going to throw a football in a spiral, you must have the proper mechanics. The doctors felt that throwing a football would be less likely to put undue stress on my arm.

Dr. Muschler gave me a stern warning, though, to pay attention to the way my arm felt. "Any little ache you feel could be a hairline fracture. If you feel the slightest pain you need to quit immediately. Don't try to keep working with that. If it's a hairline fracture, it'll set you back six weeks. But if it breaks, it sets you back a full year."

When we'd gone over the details of my training program, Dr. Bergfeld asked Dr. Muschler the big question. "Doctor, if everything goes well and Dave follows this program, when would you think, tentatively of course, he might be at full strength and ready for competition?"

That wasn't the kind of question that Muschler

ordinarily liked, so I was surprised to hear his answer. "Maybe sometime in July," he said, "if everything goes well."

I left the Cleveland Clinic with enough adrenaline to pitch the World Series.

The next day I got my brother Rick to come over after work. Rick is a year younger than I am; he works at the family business, and with his dark hair and high cheekbones looks like a movie star.

I had my football, and we took it out in the driveway. It was a cold late afternoon, and the sun had long since disappeared in the tall trees behind our house. I warned Rick not to fool around or try to throw the ball too hard, because my bone was brittle and I had to be careful. I told him to pace off thirty feet, then took the football in my hand and threw.

It felt weird. First of all, it felt strange to be throwing after so many months. Throwing something was, after all, my livelihood, the thing I did best and the thing I did most. For all those months I hadn't done it once.

It also felt weird in my shoulder. I could tell that something was missing. When the muscles tightened I could feel them, because half of my deltoid wasn't there to tighten with them. I could feel the void.

I took five short throws, and went inside. That was all the doctors allowed for starters.

By the end of January, I was engaged full-scale in daily workouts, riding the stationary bicycle, lifting weights, throwing the football three times a week at increasing distances. I felt great. After all those months of inactivity, I was elated about working up a sweat.

I also felt cooped up from the long winter. Janice and I had decided that we needed to get away. We took the kids out of school and headed south, feeling excited. It was the first real family vacation we'd ever had.

We went first to Anderson, South Carolina, where Janice's brother Randy lives. We stayed with him and his family for a couple of days, and then headed for Knoxville, Tennessee. That's where Atlee and Jenny Hammaker hang out in the off-season. Ever since we'd known them they'd been telling us about their place, way out in the middle of nowhere. They'd shown us pictures. A couple of years before, Scott and Kathy Garrelts had gone to visit for a few days and stayed two weeks. Now we were going to see for ourselves.

Outside of Knoxville I stopped at a service station and called Atlee for directions. He told me where to get off the freeway, and said he'd meet me at a certain truck stop. We pulled up at the same time. Atlee was in his pickup with a big golden retriever named Austin. We barely said hi and Atlee took off, leading the way.

We followed a series of country roads, getting farther away from people at every turn. It was rolling foothill farm country, pretty to look at even in the middle of winter with no snow. We went down a long country lane that passed a lake, and then Atlee turned left and headed straight up a hill. I looked up and said to Janice, "Look at that!"

At the top of the hill was the Hammakers' place,

a roomy, colonial-style home with white columns and a 360-degree view of the surrounding mountains. Actually, the house belongs to Jenny's parents. The Hammakers own some property down on the lake, but they haven't gotten around to building a home of their own. They live with Jenny's parents, the Johnsons, in the off-season.

It's a large, comfortable home, but we definitely filled it. Scott and Kathy had already arrived, so the four Draveckys got the last bedroom.

When I walked in, Scott was cooking some deer meat for dinner. The aroma filled the house. Everybody came out and wanted to see my scar. They admired it so much that I thought they really ought to see my leg. Because the fascia was cut open, the muscle bulges out just under the skin in a big, nasty-looking tube. I put on some shorts and did the medical fashion show.

The next day I told Scott and Atlee I'd like to throw the football a little. I warned them that the bone was brittle. They would need to take it easy and not fool around.

We got out in the front yard and started to lob the ball back and forth. It was a beautiful, clear, crisp winter's day. Pretty soon they saw that I could throw the ball as hard as they could. Atlee said, "Forget taking it easy on you, Dravecky." He started zinging the ball. From that day on, Atlee said, he knew I was going to come back. If I could throw a football as hard as he could, he knew I'd be able to pitch.

For five days we did next to nothing. Everybody wore blue jeans—or pajamas—and we sat around the fire talking. We chased kids, we did a little working out. Jenny Hammaker was nursing a new baby, and had recently fallen and broken her leg, so she couldn't move too fast. My daughter Tiffany got sick with the flu soon after we arrived and passed it on to everybody else. A lot of activity wasn't feasible. What we had going for us was *togetherness.*

It was hard staying at home when everybody else went to spring training at the end of February. I talked to Scott and Atlee often on the phone, and they complained that it wasn't the same without us. They had taken units in the same apartment complex again, but their apartments were a little farther apart, and it seemed harder to get together. They said they were missing us. We were certainly missing them.

In mid-March, about two weeks before the start of the season, I got permission to throw a baseball for the first time. I wasn't supposed to throw it hard, but at least I could throw it.

I called up Bob Stauffer, my pastor. He had been throwing the football with me. I told him to get out his glove.

Bob had played college baseball—he was a catcher—and had even been drafted, though he'd chosen to go to seminary instead. We headed for Canfield High School, which has a big gym. With the football, I had Bob gradually work back to a distance of about ninety feet—a good, long toss which I was able to make without any trouble. I even tried some tosses sitting in a chair, and was able to get plenty on it. My arm felt great. The time for throwing the baseball had come.

COMEBACK

We got our gloves, stepped off sixty feet or so, and began. My first toss went straight into the floor about twenty-five feet in front of me. It bounced and hit Bob on the shin. He laughed, held his leg, and threw the ball back to me.

I was wild. That's an unfamiliar feeling for me, as a control pitcher. I was bouncing the ball off the bleachers, off the walls, off nearly everything. I wasn't alarmed about it. I just had forgotten how to throw a ball. Everything was out of sync.

What mattered to me was the feeling of holding that ball and letting it go. I wanted to throw it through a wall. Of course, that was my adrenaline talking. My mind said I'd be lucky to get it to the wall.

But though the arm was weak, the feeling was strong. Oh, sure, we were just in a gym, playing catch in front of a dozen curious high school kids. But I knew I wasn't all that far from throwing in a live game. I wanted to get back between the lines.

Hitting the Wall

I was so anxious to start that I went to Arizona for the last two days of spring training, even though most of the team had left town for exhibition games in New Orleans. I was just happy to put on spikes and walk onto a baseball diamond. I found Atlee, played a little catch, and did some running under the blue Arizona sky. A few players and coaches were around. Everybody who saw me throw was amazed. They were expecting some kind of altered, cockeyed delivery. My motion was the same as ever.

I felt great. For the first time in a year I had no pain. And I was in baseball land again. I told everybody who would listen that I was coming back. I told them I would pitch before the summer was up.

It felt even better to arrive in San Francisco and walk into the clubhouse at Candlestick Park, the Giants' stadium. The Giants' quarters are not about to appear in *Architectural Digest*. They feature bright orange carpet underfoot (orange and black are the Giants' colors) and white-painted industrial-strength pipe overhead. The "lockers" are open-air partitions about four feet wide, painted black and white. It could be the locker room at a Chrysler plant. But for six months of the year it's my home away from home, and it felt great to get back.

I was made to feel welcome immediately. Left-fielder Kevin Mitchell examined my arm and said, "Man, you look like Jaws took a bite out of you." Mike Krukow, a fellow pitcher, looked over my body and summed it up: "You're certainly no day at the beach." In about sixty seconds I felt like I'd never been gone. I don't know why ballplayers abuse each other, but at least they are equal-opportunity abusers. You walk in the door, you take your abuse like everybody else.

The next day I drove down to see Larry Brown, the Giants' physical therapist. I was feeling like a living miracle. The thought occurred to me: I've had a year and a half of nearly total rest. Maybe my pitching career will be given an extended life. Physically, I've always been a late developer. They called me Lady Schick in college, because I still hardly needed to shave. Maybe I'll get old late too. Maybe I'll be pitching into my forties, like Tommy John or Rick Reuschel.

Larry Brown's clinic is located in Palo Alto, in a crowded neighborhood mixing apartments, old homes, and small businesses. Dr. Campbell, the team's physician, has his offices downstairs in the same building.

Larry and I met in the main therapy room, a bare chamber with undecorated beige walls and a scattering of weight machines. Larry is soft-spoken but extremely intense. He doesn't shout and he doesn't kid around. He takes his work seriously. We knew each other well, since he had worked with me during most of the previous season, trying to help me get over my sore shoulder. With Larry I knew I was working with the best, somebody who could be tough where I needed it. He understood exactly what I was capable of doing, and he would expect all of it.

We sat down on one of the training tables and got right down to business, talking through all that had happened to me since my operation. Larry let the air out of my balloon right away. He's not the kind of guy who pats you on the back and tells you how great you are, and he didn't seem impressed by what I'd accomplished. What impressed Larry was the amount of work I would have to do. Knowing what the doctors had done to my arm, and understanding the physiological implications, he couldn't see much reason for excitement. What he saw ahead was sweat, and more sweat.

"Dave," Larry said, "you need to think like a prize fighter who's got six weeks to prepare for the biggest match of his life. Only instead of a six-million-dollar prize, you're training to get a chance to pitch again. You're going to work like you've never worked before. You'll have to push yourself each day as though you'll never get a second chance."

Larry wasn't trying to psych me up. He was warning me. He said he wanted to work with me five days a week. Having worked with Larry before, I wasn't thrilled. Larry's workouts are the toughest I've ever been through.

I had worn workout clothes, expecting that we

would get started. Larry did not disappoint me. To test my strength, he put me through a series of arm exercises. He would hold my left wrist or elbow, and I'd push against him in a particular direction—across my body, or out from my side, for example—through several repetitions. Larry felt that he could evaluate my strength better in this hands-on way than through any machine testing.

In some areas he found I had no strength at all. He would be pushing against my arm and telling me, "Hold it, Dave. Hold it there."

"That's all there is, Larry," I said with a grunt, and dropped my arm.

After the workout Larry sat me down again. He said that we had a rough road ahead—even rougher than he'd anticipated. He thought I might have to change my delivery. Without the deltoid muscle to hold my shoulder together, my arm could fly right out of its socket. A shorter-armed delivery would put less torque on my arm when I released the ball.

In any case, my arm was really weak. If I was going to pitch a baseball, the other muscles in the shoulder girdle would have to be strong enough to compensate for the deltoid's absence. I had a long, long way to go.

I got home and dumped myself in the living room of our apartment. When you're flying high you can land hard. I did. I didn't want to talk, not even to Janice. When I filled her in briefly on what had happened, she was sobered as well.

Until that day, nobody had said a discouraging word. The doctors had been awed at my progress.

My teammates were amazed when they saw me throw. But Larry, who knew my arm, and who understood the mechanics of throwing the baseball as well as anybody, had dumped cold water all over me. I was looking at grueling work for weeks and months to come, and Larry didn't seem very optimistic about my chances for success.

I couldn't discount his opinion. I'd felt what he'd felt when he took me through the exercises. I respected Larry tremendously. If anybody could evaluate my prospects, he could.

I hated the idea of messing with my delivery. I'd needed all these years to gain an understanding of my mechanics, to feel that I could adjust in just a pitch or two. I didn't want to fool with that. It would be like trying to learn to pitch right-handed.

Luckily for me, one of the *Rocky* movies came on that night, and Janice gave me permission to watch it. I say "permission" because she hates violent TV. But she saw how down I was, and she relented. I was in my glory, watching Rocky destroy the bad guys. It gave me a lift.

The next morning I drove down the Bayshore freeway to see Larry again. He met me in his white shirt and dark slacks, his horn-rimmed glasses and his all-business manner. I got on the table and we began going through sets of manual-resistance exercises, just as we had the day before. Soon Larry stopped. I thought I knew why. Just as before, I couldn't sustain the exercises.

"Let's let it go at that," Larry said in a leaden voice. "There's no use in pushing it beyond what you can do. Let's just go out and throw and see how that feels."

From what he had seen of my arm, Larry couldn't have been expecting much. He probably thought I'd shot-put the ball to him. We got our gloves and went out into the clinic's small, crowded parking lot. I hadn't thrown three times before Larry stopped.

"How are you doing that?" he asked. His tone was completely changed. "You shouldn't be able to throw that way."

It wasn't how hard I was throwing, it was the fact that my delivery was unchanged. Since I was missing most of a major arm muscle, he'd assumed that my delivery would be massively affected.

I walked over to him, my glove under my arm. "Larry, I think you understand where I'm coming from. As far as I'm concerned, this has all been a miracle of God."

Larry said, with that puzzled look on his face, "There's no other way to explain it as far as I'm concerned." We went back to throwing.

When we were done we talked again. Larry's attitude was different. He seemed much more confident. "All right, let's go," he said. "We're going to get you going no matter what. Your delivery looks fine. It won't need much change, if any. Let's just get you strong and see where that takes us."

Every morning, starting about nine o'clock, I did forty-five minutes of exercises with Larry. Soon, as I gained strength, we added routines with weights. Three days a week I threw the ball. Every day I did an aerobic workout on the stationary bike.

It was a tough day's work. Oftentimes others

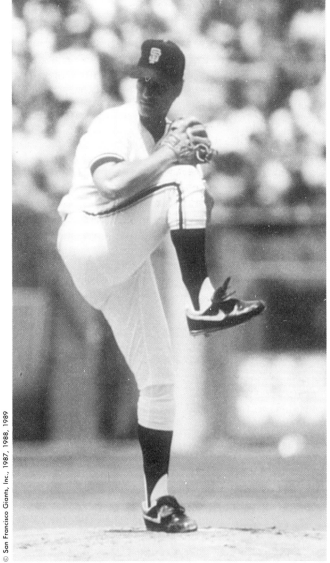

© San Francisco Giants, Inc., 1987, 1988, 1989

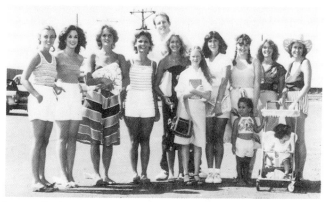

Byron Ballard, who was instru-
mental in my new interest and
commitment to Christianity, is
shown here with some of the
wives and kids of my Amarillo
teammates.

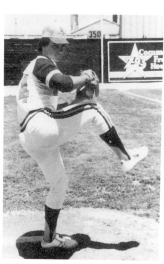

Pitching in Amarillo

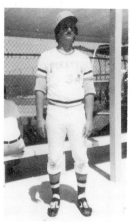

My first spring training in the pros

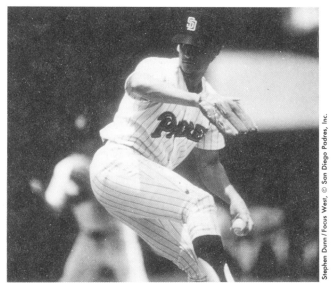

Stephen Dunn / Focus West, © San Diego Padres, Inc.

My first stop in the majors was with the San Diego Padres.

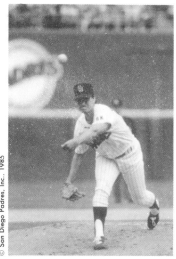

© San Diego Padres, Inc., 1985

I spent six years in San Diego from 1981-1987, and pitched in the 1984 National League Championship Series (N.L.C.S.) and the World Series for the Padres.

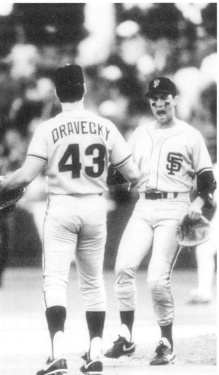

© San Francisco Giants, Inc., 1987, 1988, 1989

In July 1987 I was traded to the San Francisco Giants who were vying for the pennant. Will Clark was the first to congratulate me after my victory in game two of the N.L.C.S.

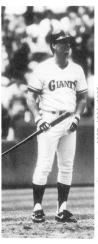

© San Francisco Giants, Inc., 1987, 1988, 1989

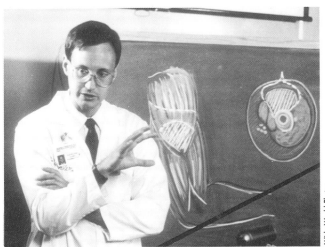

Wide World Photos

Less than a year after the euphoria of playing in a league championship series had subsided, I faced the harsh reality of surgery to remove a lump that had become more than just a "nuisance."

Above—Dr. Muschler describes the operation for the media. Removing the cancerous tumor required removal of 50% of my deltoid muscle.

Right—Little did I know that the surgery and rehabilitation procedures in the months leading up to and including my return to the big leagues would put me in the spotlight with the media.

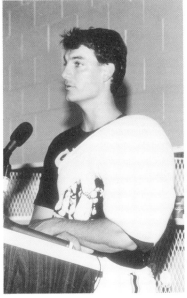

Mickey Pfleger / Sports Illustrated / © Time Inc.

August 10, 1989—In the words of my manager, Roger Craig, "Today we're going to witness a miracle." And in an amazing display of God's grace, we did! According to the prognosis following surgery, I wasn't supposed to be able to take my wallet out of my pocket.... Instead, in less than a year, I was back pitching in the majors against the Cincinnati Reds.

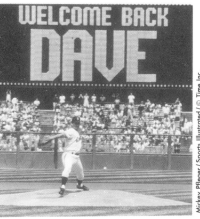

Mickey Pfleger / Sports Illustrated / © Time Inc.

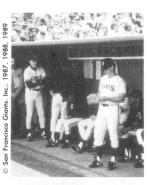

© San Francisco Giants, Inc., 1987, 1988, 1989

For me, for Janice, for most everyone watching the game that day, the feeling was electric. It was hard enough concentrating on the game during warm-ups in the bull pen, but when they flashed the message on the giant scoreboard and the crowd roared...I was overcome with emotion.

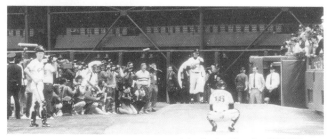

© San Francisco Giants, Inc., 1987, 1988, 1989

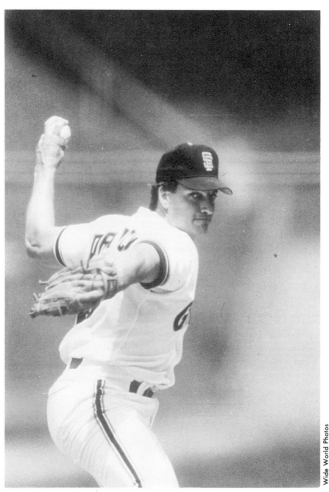

Wide World Photos

With all the standing ovations I received during my "Comeback Game," my hat came off in gratitude more than once. The toughest part was making that first pitch, but after saying a brief prayer right there on the mound, I sensed an unusual peace. Then the miracle was underway.

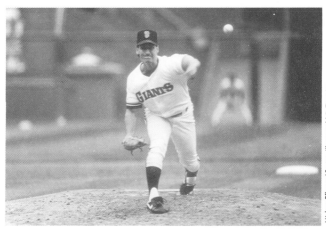

Mickey Pfleger / Sports Illustrated / © Time Inc.

The first batter, Luis Quinones, popped out to center field on a full count and the cheers rained down. From then on through seven innings it was just a picture: Terry Kennedy and me playing catch, as though nobody else was around. I had my stuff and even my defensive fielding held up.

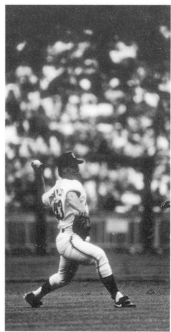

© San Francisco Giants, Inc., 1987, 1988, 1989

Roger Craig pulled me in the bottom of the eighth since I had begun to struggle in the top of that inning. But you can be sure I didn't head to the showers. Our stopper, Steve "Bedrock" Bedrosian, faced only three batters, and he had fire. Just like that, the game was over.

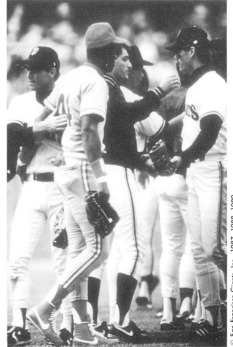

© San Francisco Giants, Inc., 1987, 1988, 1989

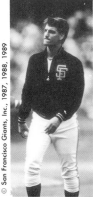

© San Francisco Giants, Inc., 1987, 1988, 1989

I was on my feet before the last swinging strike. I ran out toward the mound and the celebration began. Even the Cincinnati players offered their congratulations. The fans were still cheering, yelling as though they'd never stop, even as I walked off the field.

Alex Vlahos is a special part of my story. He's a little boy with leukemia whom I'd visited in June of 1989 at Stanford Children's Hospital. During my "Comeback Game," a local radio station, KNBR, organized a fund-raising drive for Alex based on every pitch I threw. The money went to *Life-Savers Foundation* to help find a donor for a bone marrow transplant for Alex.

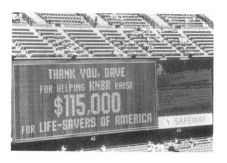

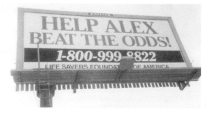

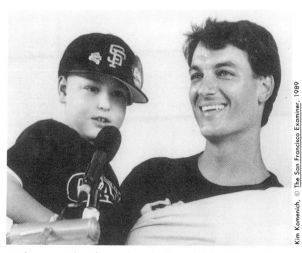

Kim Komenich, © <u>The San Francisco Examiner</u>, 1989

When I met Alex afterwards I asked him what he felt about the game. His simple response was beautiful—"Uh, you did good."

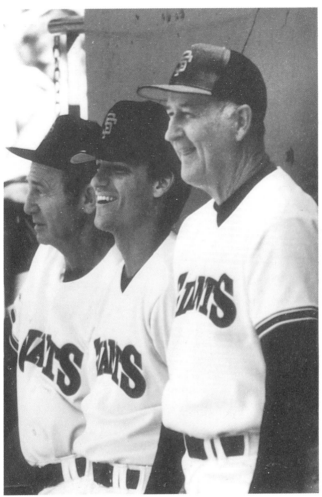

Two of the many people in the Giants' organization who believed in me
and gave me a chance to come back were my pitching coach, Norm
Sherry (left), and our manager, Roger Craig (right). Roger said that in all
the decades he'd played and coached, he'd never seen so much emotion
at a game.

August 15, 1989—
Five days after the comeback game, I was scheduled to pitch in Montreal. Things seemed much more settled in this "away" game and I was glad. I was back to normal and it was a normal game. That is until the sixth inning. . . .

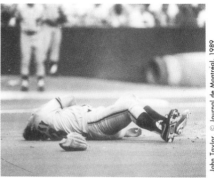

John Taylor, © Journal de Montréal, 1989

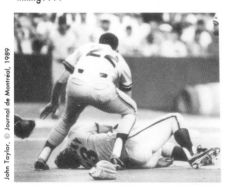

John Taylor, © Journal de Montréal, 1989

On the first pitch to Tim Raines my world was shattered again. I felt as though my arm had separated from my body and was sailing off toward home plate. The pain was incredible.

Will Clark was the first to reach me as I was writhing and grunting, trying to get my breath. As they wheeled me off, I knew I'd broken my arm.

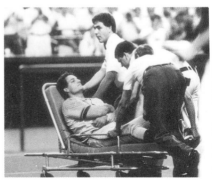

John Taylor, © Journal de Montréal, 1989

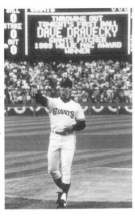

© San Francisco Giants, Inc., 1987, 1988, 1989

Once again, we found ourselves competing for the National League pennant. Only this time the only pitch I was able to throw was a ceremonial "first pitch" prior to game 3.

All my son, Jonathan, and I could do during the National League Championship Series was watch practice from the stands.

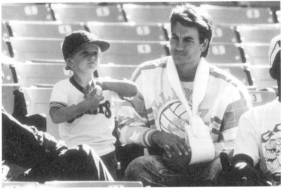

Wide World Photos

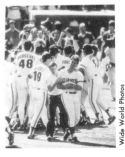

Wide World Photos

We won the pennant in five games and I wasn't about to miss the celebration. Perhaps I should have. In the mound melee, I broke my arm again....

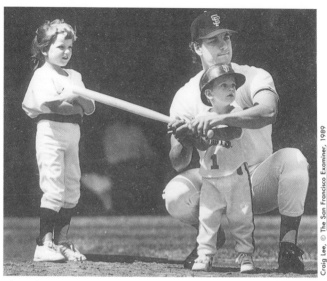

Craig Lee, © The San Francisco Examiner, 1989

I love playing ball with my children, Tiffany and Jonathan.

One of the greatest gifts I enjoy is family. God has blessed Janice and me with rich heritages and a wonderful opportunity to build a legacy of faith into our own children. One valuable lesson I've learned in the past few years is how important it is to keep a balanced perspective on life. In the long run, family has to be a top priority.

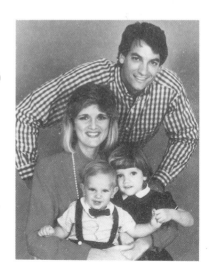

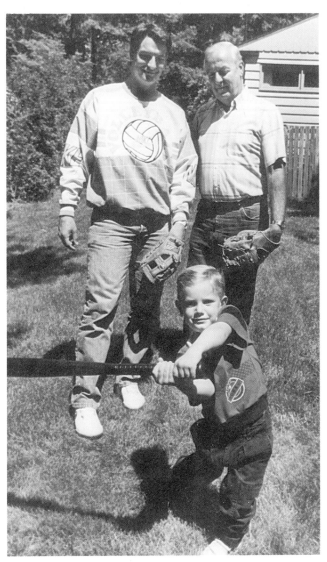

Three generations of Draveckys—me, Dad, and Jonathan

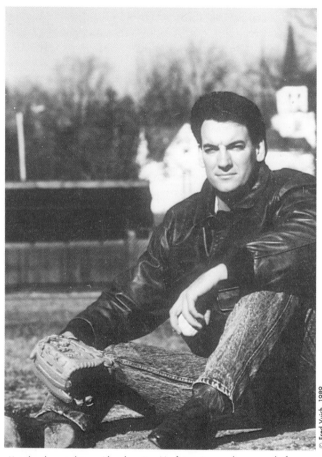

© Fred Vuich, 1989

I'm clearly not done with adversity. My future is as unknown as before. All I can say for certain is that I'm done playing baseball.

When I think back on my career, I do so with a big, fat smile on my face. How could I feel anything else?

I'm one of the fortunate few who was able to realize the dream of playing in the major leagues. I got to play with the big boys. And for that, I'm grateful.

who were getting therapy would stop by and look at what we were doing. I can remember them commenting, "Boy, I'm glad you're not working like that on me, Larry."

Typically I'd get home from the clinic about one in the afternoon, absolutely exhausted. For at least an hour I'd sink into my chair and say nothing. If anybody disturbed me I'd be extremely grumpy.

When the team was in town—I didn't travel with them through April and May—I went out to the ballpark in the afternoon for the team workout. I'd throw and do my exercise routine there. Everybody on the team was extremely encouraging. My buddies all said they were rooting for me. They said they knew I was going to make it back.

By the end of April, though, I was beginning to worry. I told Janice, "I'm not getting anywhere. I'm on a plateau."

My arm had gained strength at a very rapid pace, my stamina was tremendously increased, but it wasn't translating to throwing the ball. I felt as though my arm was dead. It just followed obediently through the motion of throwing. There was no snap to it, no vitality. I tried to fire the ball, but I found nothing there.

At the ballpark everybody was rooting me on, and I didn't see any point in telling them they were wasting their breath. But in private, talking to Janice and Larry Brown, I admitted that I was concerned. For the first time I began seriously questioning the possibility of a comeback.

I appreciate that Larry is a realist. When you talk to Larry, you get the unvarnished facts. I told him what I was feeling, and he didn't try to gloss over it. He didn't know how to interpret what was happening. I was missing a major arm muscle. Nobody had ever tried to pitch without a deltoid. Maybe I was feeling the physiological fact: There *was* nothing there.

Then, after two weeks on that plateau, my arm began to hurt. The pain was not where the tumor had been removed, but in the back of my shoulder. At first it was just a minor stiffness, but soon I'd make a few pitches and feel the pain build.

In previous years I would have tried to tough it out, but Larry had emphasized that I had to be honest with him about anything I was feeling. He and the doctors needed to know.

Larry had me cut back on the throwing, to see whether a lighter load would help. He suspected that perhaps fatigue was contributing to my problems. I never pushed it; when my arm hurt, I quit throwing. But rest didn't seem to make any difference. I began to wonder whether I'd ever really recovered from my 1988 arm troubles.

The pain grew worse. Larry gave me a couple of days off, to see whether that would help, but when I tried to throw again the pain was terrible.

Instead of the cheery, encouraging comments I'd been hearing from my teammates, I began to get a lot of sympathetic looks. Roger Craig would pass by and ask me how it was going, but looking at the mournful expression on his face I didn't think he wanted an honest answer.

Strength wasn't the problem. I was bench pressing more weight than I had in my whole life. The problem was that I couldn't throw.

Larry drove up to watch me at the ballpark a

couple of times. The first time I threw, things went fairly well. My shoulder was sore, but I was able to make pitches. The next time, a couple of days later, my shoulder felt as though somebody had hammered a six-penny nail into it. I tried to work through the pain for a few tosses, but my arm just tightened up more. I had to quit. Feeling frustrated, wondering whether it had all been useless, I told Larry I couldn't go on. I had hit the wall.

Two days later, I went into the outfield to shag balls and throw them back into the infield—just lazy, easy tosses. But my shoulder was too painful to bear. The ball would loop eighty feet or so and bury itself in the grass. My arm felt paralyzed with pain. I simply could not throw.

That evening I met with Dr. Campbell, and he recommended that I shut down my workouts completely. They weren't helping. He suggested that I go down to Larry's clinic three times a week for an ultrasound treatment, and then ice down the arm. That would be it. No exercise, no nothing. Only time would tell whether I could ever throw again.

For me, waiting is much harder than any amount of work. I was in a fog emotionally. Teammates were feeling sorry for me. I was feeling sorry for myself. I went up to Atlee one day and said, "If I have to retire, Atlee, will you still be my friend? Will you still invite me to Tennessee?"

"What are you talking about retirement for?" Atlee said. "You're not ready for that."

I wasn't so sure. Nick and Lee Hoslag, whose fitness center I'd used for workouts in San Diego, came up to visit on their anniversary. They're close friends, people I respect. They were strongly urging me to give it up.

"What are you trying to prove, Dave?" Nick asked. "Do you realize that the stress of throwing can aggravate the cancer cells, if any were left in there? Why would you keep pushing your career when it involves that kind of risk? Don't you know you have a family to care for?"

I didn't have any answer for him. I wasn't really communicating very well, even with Janice. I wasn't communicating very well with myself.

Janice has never been fond of the way baseball affects our family life. She's a planner, and the uncertainty of our life just then was driving her crazy. She worried about what I was doing to my arm. Was I risking a recurrence of cancer for a comeback that could never be? Yet at the same time she wondered: Why would God have opened so many doors only to slam this one closed? When so many miraculous things had occurred, should we be quick to give up? Janice went back and forth. She didn't know. Neither did I.

Nonetheless, Janice asked me to request a special favor from the team. "See if we can go along on the road trip. See if they'll let you go as a vacation, just for old time's sake."

The Giants have a provision whereby players can take their families along for two road trips during the year. These are usually a lot of fun, since you stay in fancy hotels and have a chance to see some of the country with your wife and kids. We'd looked forward to a trip that would pass through

Pittsburgh. We'd planned to stay at our home in Youngstown for a few days.

The trip was due to begin July 2. According to Dr. Muschler's original schedule, I should have been preparing for a pitching assignment about then. But at the beginning of June, as I rested and wondered what my future would be, traveling with the team was out of the picture. It might never enter the picture again, if my arm kept hurting. Janice thought the trip might be our last chance. She wanted the children to have the experience. She was building memories.

I wasn't quite ready to build memories. It would have been simpler, I knew, to take that approach. If this was to be the end of my career, fine. Make your plans. Take your final trips. Say your good-byes. But was that realistic? Nobody really knew. Nobody had ever gone through what I was going through. There wasn't any predictable pattern, because mine was the first case ever.

My uncertainty came to a head one day after Janice took a call from the athletic director of a state university in the Midwest. He told her he was interested in discussing a coaching job with me.

To Janice, the call was heaven sent. She wrote down the number and told me about it when I came home. We had often talked about how much I'd like coaching at a college level.

I didn't say much. I put the number aside and said I'd call, but I didn't. I wasn't entirely clear myself on why. I just knew I wasn't ready.

Janice reminded me that I was to call back. I put her off. The next day she reminded me again.

"Don't you want to call him? I really think you should call him."

I put her off again. The third day she was still reminding me. Or call it nagging. "David, I really don't understand why you're not calling him. Why don't you at least talk to the man?"

Then, suddenly, I knew how I felt.

I gave her a hard look. "Don't count me out yet," I said.

I knew she'd be hurt. Janice has always been my biggest supporter. Not necessarily my biggest fan, but always my biggest supporter. There's a difference. Janice rooted for me all the way. She rooted for me because baseball was my chosen career—not because baseball, apart from me, mattered all that much.

When we were in the minor leagues and somebody would say that I wasn't going to make it, she never got terribly upset. She believed I would make it in the majors if I got the chance. But her accountant's mind told her I might very well not get the chance. We knew plenty of good players who, because of injuries or timing, never did. Janice's response was always, "Well, if that's so, it's fine with me. I didn't marry him for baseball."

My mom didn't quite see eye to eye with Janice on that. They dearly love each other, but on the subject of my life in baseball they have their differences. My mom has always been my supporter, and also my fan. It mattered to her that I made it in baseball. She didn't understand why it didn't ultimately matter to Janice.

When I'd returned to San Francisco after winning the 1988 opening-day game in Los Angeles, my mom and Janice had been sitting together in the stands for the Giants' home opener. When the team was introduced to the fans, I got a standing ovation. My mom turned to Janice and said, "And you thought he'd never make it."

That was in both my mind and Janice's when I said, "Don't count me out yet."

But there was more to my statement. All winter, when I'd been working out and gaining strength day by day, I'd told people that I'd explore every avenue and exhaust every last ounce of energy to make a comeback. If I'd done everything possible, and I was truly unable to play again, I could accept the end of my baseball career with grace.

I didn't believe I'd reached that point yet. And truthfully, neither did Janice.

15

Air It Out

FOR one month I did nothing but pedal the stationary bike. I showed up at practice, I went to the games, I put on a uniform—but I couldn't even play catch. I didn't feel as though I was a real baseball player. I felt like a ghost. I was caught in between two worlds, the world of baseball and the "real" world outside—and I didn't know which I was headed toward.

The team was doing well, staying at the top of their division. They played incredible cliff-hanging games. They lost some dreadfully, and they won some stunningly. Watching the Giants must have been hard on cardiac patients.

My buddy Scott Garrelts, who had suffered through spring training as a would-be stopper, had converted to a starter and was performing brilliantly. Kevin Mitchell was hitting home runs at a Babe-Ruth pace. Rick Reuschel, on the verge of forty, was putting on a pitching clinic every time he started. Will Clark was rapping the ball every which direction, his eyes glittering and his fists clenched as he rounded first base again and again.

All this meant that the Giants weren't spending a lot of time thinking about Dave Dravecky. When you're hurt and the team's doing poorly, people tend to say, "If only you were healthy." They had said that in 1988. But when you're hurt and the team is in first place, people tend to forget you. Obviously you're not the crucial missing ingredient.

Rick Reuschel came up to me one day. Big Daddy, as he's called, rarely has much to say, but when he talks I listen.

"Dave," he said, "I know what it's like to come back from injuries. There are times when you're sure you're not getting anywhere. You just have to be patient. If you keep working, you can slowly build past those obstacles and reach the next level. Don't give up. Be patient."

But patience doesn't come easily for me. I was tired of waiting. I wanted to move, in whatever direction.

During the second week in June, Larry Brown told me we needed to have a conference. My month of rest was over. He wanted to discuss my future plans.

When I got to the clinic I was honest with Larry. We sat down on a training table, and I told him, "You know, Larry, considering the fatigue you and Dr. Campbell have talked about, I wonder whether we ought to cut back on the workouts. Maybe we should just emphasize throwing the ball." I said it somewhat uncertainly, remembering Larry's reference to training like a prize fighter.

I was surprised when Larry said he had similar thoughts. He had just come upstairs from talking over my situation with Dr. Campbell. They had agreed that the workouts had taken me as far as they should go.

"To be perfectly honest with you, Dave, you shouldn't be able to do what you're doing. I don't understand how it's happening. If you come back and pitch, it's just a miracle.

"So you might as well take your chances. Go ahead and throw. See what you're capable of doing and what you're not capable of doing. We've done everything that we can for you. Your arm is strong now. You just have to see what's possible."

He did ask that I come in three times a week, so he could check my progress. But he was setting me free. I could prepare in my normal way, as a baseball player rather than as a patient in recovery.

Larry didn't tell me that all would be well. He was simply saying that therapy had nothing more to offer me. I could run my own life.

It unnerved me a bit, after I walked out of the clinic and began my drive home. During rehabilitation, you can easily become dependent on direction from doctors and therapists. It's as though someone else knows your body better than you do. You're afraid to try things on your own. You lose trust in your judgment.

Going on my own was like throwing away a crutch that I'd been using for months. I wasn't sure that I could walk without it.

By the time I pulled into my driveway, though, my mind had shifted into a positive mode. I was thinking about throwing again. At least my future would become clear on the field.

* * *

Air It Out

All you have to do is pick up a baseball. It begs to you: Throw me. If you took a year to design an object to hurl, you'd end up with that little spheroid: small enough to nestle in your fingers but big enough to have some heft, lighter than a rock but heavier than a hunk of wood. Its even, neat stitching, laced into the leather's slippery white surface, gives your fingers a purchase. A baseball was made to throw. It's almost irresistible.

When you've held baseballs by the thousands, you can detect the tiniest variation. They may all say, "Official size and weight," but some are a fraction bigger, some a bit smaller. Carpenters talk about the differences in hammers. Pitchers talk about the differences in baseballs.

I have small hands which, by the way, saved me from Roger Craig's drive to teach every Giant pitcher—every pitcher in the universe, it seemed at times—the split-finger fastball. I can't spread my fingers wide enough to hold a baseball between them.

Because I have small hands, I particularly like small baseballs. The big ones feel like grapefruits to me—oversized and soft. The little ones feel like BBs. I can often tell whether the baseball is too big as I watch it fly from the umpire's hand to my mitt. Sometimes I catch a new ball and immediately throw it back. I want small ones, tightly wrapped with nice firm seams. When you have a real pill, you feel like you can throw it one hundred miles an hour.

Oftentimes in the dugout we go through the ball bag, checking out the balls to see how they feel. When we hit a good one, we pull it out and hand it around. "Hey, here's a real pearl. Feel this one." Or when we're out shagging flies during practice, we'll find a pearl. It goes right into the back pocket. You collect good ones and use them during the winter.

I was anxious to hurl those little pills again, but I was also unsure. The first time I threw after my month of rest, I worked carefully, tentatively, feeling for the pain in the back of my shoulder. There was some soreness, though nothing profound. Uncertainty kept me from pressing too hard.

I took a day off and threw again. This time the pain was unmistakable. I went home in a gloom. "It's back," I told Janice softly. "My shoulder is hurting again. I don't think I'm going to be able to throw."

It wasn't that the pain was yet so terrible. But I felt it coming, and I knew where it led.

The next day I told Atlee that my arm was hurting, that I couldn't throw. We were out in right field, shagging fly balls under the afternoon sun. Atlee wouldn't accept what I said. He said, "Come on, Dave. Let's play some catch."

"I don't know, Atlee. I think I'd better not."

"Hey," Atlee replied. "What have you got to lose? You've done your therapy. Your arm is strong. David, the time has come. Don't baby it any more. Let it rip. If it goes, it goes."

He insisted, and I let him talk me into it. We started throwing the ball back and forth. I threw gingerly, cautiously. My shoulder felt okay. The longer I threw, the better I felt.

I told Atlee that it was feeling pretty good.

"All right," he said. "Let's throw through some

of that pain. Just work through it. Let's air this baby out."

He backed up and we began to throw hard. The ball went zipping back and forth, burrowing through the air like a bullet. I couldn't help enjoying myself. And Dr. Atlee's therapy worked. I wasn't hurting. I was really throwing. I wasn't ready to go up against Nolan Ryan, but my arm felt different. It had some life to it.

When Janice saw me come in the door that day, she knew immediately that something had changed. After a month standing still, I was moving again.

I'll always be grateful to Atlee for urging me to air it out. He knew that I was tentative, afraid of the pain. He sensed that the time had come to give it everything. That's a tough call. Sometimes you have to be patient and careful. But there's a time, too, when you have to let caution be blown to bits. You have to begin behaving like your normal self.

After that I played catch with Atlee every day. We played long toss, where you stand far apart in the outfield and make long, arcing, outfielder's throws. We played short toss, putting sizzle on each throw like a pitcher or an infielder. The pain receded. My arm was alive.

Within a few days I began thinking that I should try throwing from the mound. I went to the bull pen and threw to a catcher for ten minutes, not trying to do anything fancy, just getting the feel of pitching from the rubber again. The next day I went for fifteen minutes, and felt great.

Norm Sherry, our pitching coach, was watching.

He suggested that I throw batting practice. The next day, June 19, I did. That was another step forward, pitching with a batter at the plate. Norm or Roger Craig stood behind me, watching my delivery from behind a screen. The first time, I threw for fifteen minutes. Toward the end I was tired, but it was a healthy kind of fatigue, and there was very little soreness afterward.

I was gaining momentum.

I went on the road with the team for the first time, to San Diego and Houston. I would throw batting practice and take two days of rest, or else throw on the sidelines and take one day of rest. By the time we got back to San Francisco I was throwing thirty minutes of batting practice. A lot of our coaches won't do that. That's a lot of pitches.

I wasn't trying to throw at game speed, of course. I was just getting my rhythm, getting the feeling of pitching again. I was trying to hit some spots with my location. Atlee would sometimes stand behind the screen with the coaches, watching me throw. Other guys on the team would stop by and observe for a while. I can remember Robby Thompson, our second baseman, walking away shaking his head. "It's amazing," he said.

On July 2 we left for Pittsburgh. This was the family trip that I'd begged to go on for old time's sake. We stayed at our house in Youngstown for the three games in Pittsburgh—Janice and I and our kids, Atlee and Jenny Hammaker and theirs. We'd just had a lawn put in, and the genuine Midwest summer days felt terrific—hot and humid, unlike the chilly San Francisco summer weather. Atlee and I had an hour and a half commute to the Pittsburgh stadium each day, but they were pleasant drives on back-country roads. We talked nonstop. Janice and Jenny stayed home and did the same.

On Thursday, July 6, I took off and drove up to the Cleveland Clinic. I had another MRI done and saw Dr. Muschler. He checked several lumps in my arm, including a large one that had filled in the gap where my tumor had been removed. Muschler told me this lump might be a recurrence of the tumor, but he said it was too soon to tell. It could be scar tissue. It would be months before we would know.

That shook me a little, but I didn't spend much time worrying about it. We were going on to St. Louis, where the coaches had scheduled a simulated game for me on July 8—my first taste of genuine pitching.

A simulated game is as close to a real game as you can make it. The hitters are from your own team, but they are trying to make you look bad. You are trying to make them look bad. You have fielders behind you. You have to hold runners on, and cover bases. You make plays. It's completely different from batting practice, where you just lay each pitch in there to be hit. It's a *real* test.

That Saturday afternoon the temperature was 103 degrees on the St. Louis Cardinals' carpet, and the humidity made you feel that you couldn't get any wetter *in* the Mississippi River than you were on its banks. I felt sluggish. So did everybody else.

It's usually hard to get players for simulated games. Since it means coming to the ballpark an hour and a half early, nobody is very excited to have a chance to participate, especially on days when the air is so thick you want to choke on it. Generally the coaches recruit pitchers to play the field, and shanghai reserves and utility players to hit. Five or six guys take turns at the plate.

This time the coaches didn't have any trouble recruiting, though. I wasn't the only one feeling excited about my comeback. There were a lot of guys standing around to see how I was doing.

In a simulated game you throw a certain number of pitches per inning. For me it was twenty. The coaches will sometimes let you finish a batter, but more often they'll stop you in the middle of the at-bat, no matter what the count. You take a break for five minutes, while a coach throws batting practice. During that interval you can talk to the coaches, and see how fast the speed gun says you threw. Then you go out for twenty more pitches.

There's usually a screen set up behind home plate, so the coaches and the guy running the speed gun can watch from close range. There's no umpire, so the catcher calls balls and strikes. And there's a noticeable lack of effort when guys run the bases. (Except when someone hits a home run. Then, naturally, the full parade is laid on.)

In St. Louis I threw three innings, for a total of sixty pitches. That might be the equivalent of five or six innings in a real game. I wasn't really delighted with the results. Watching from the stands, Janice asked Scott Garrelts, "Is he okay? He's getting roped."

Scotty told her not to worry—you don't think about results in your first simulated game. The main thing is to get the rhythm of a real game. I was able to put the ball where I wanted it most of the time. My fastball got up to eighty-two or eighty-three miles per hour, which was not bad. At my best it usually tops out at eighty-eight.

My slider didn't have much break on it, but that didn't surprise me. It was the same every spring. For me, this was like spring training. The difference was that we were locked in a pennant race, and our pitching staff was suffering from a wide variety of injuries. They needed me out there. And, caught up in the momentum of the pennant race, I wanted to be out there contributing.

We returned home for the All-Star break, after which I pitched a second simulated game while the Pittsburgh Pirates were in town. I threw better and felt stronger. My fastball had a little more pop on it, and I began to get a few guys out.

I was then scheduled to throw a five-inning simulated game. The date was July 18, just over a month from the time when Atlee had convinced me to take a chance and air it out. Reporters were talking with me. Teammates were excited. Nobody could believe how far I had come. Not even me. I was moving full speed ahead.

As bad as the nights can be in Candlestick Park, when the cold fog blows in on a swirling wind, the summer afternoons are unbeatable. Looking up at a bright blue sky, visitors would have a hard time believing that an evening hurricane is about to blast in.

My simulated game fell on that kind of day. Five innings meant that I would be throwing one hundred pitches. That's equivalent to a good, full-game effort. I was still trying to focus on one day at a time, but by this point the light at the end of the tunnel was blinding.

The sun was warm on my shoulders, and rock music was blaring out over the field. A scattering of coaches and players were there to watch. I was hitting spots, I was throwing crisp pitches. And most of the time I was getting guys out.

Only one thing was missing. I was still a little tentative. It probably would not have been visible to anyone but another pitcher or a pitching coach. But they knew: I was still slightly afraid.

When I went out to pitch the last inning, Norm Sherry came over to me. "Dave," he said, "the last five or six pitches, just let it go. Air it out. Let's see what you can do."

So when I got down to the last few pitches, and was beginning to feel the fatigue of throwing, I told the batter that I was going to let some fastballs rip.

"Be careful," I said. I wasn't sure just where they were headed.

I wound up and let the ball go. *Boom!* Lo and behold, it went over the plate. More importantly, my arm did not pop off and roll toward first base. When I had thrown my one hundredth pitch Norm called a halt, and I jogged over to the screen.

"How fast was I?" I asked.

"You got up to eighty-five."

"Fantastic!" That was only three miles per hour less than my norm. "I'm fired up now!"

I turned to Norm Sherry. "Hey, Norm, what do you think? I'm ready for some competition! I want to go down to Phoenix and get some guys out!"

Up Through the Minor Leagues

I'D wanted to go straight to Phoenix for my rehabilitation with our Triple-A team. But Al Rosen, the general manager of the Giants, surprised me by sending me to San Jose, instead. San Jose is an A-level team, composed mostly of kids only a year or two out of school.

These kids worried me plenty. I had heard horror stories. If you get beat at the Triple-A level, that's respectable, but if you get beat by A-level kids, the management regards that as a problem. Yet these guys are free swingers. I'm a finesse pitcher, who gets people out by fooling them, not blowing them away. These kids might not know enough to be fooled.

Nevertheless, five days after my last simulated game Nick Glass picked me up to drive to Stockton. The San Jose Giants were playing there, and I was the scheduled pitcher.

I locked the door on an empty apartment. On Wednesday, Janice had taken the kids home to Youngstown, Ohio. It was a classic mix-up. We had thought I would be either with the Giants on a two-week road trip, or else sent directly to Phoenix. Janice didn't want to be trapped with the kids

in a Phoenix hotel room while the temperature outside was 120 degrees. As it turned out, the Giants
chose a third option—nearby San Jose. I slept at
home during the entire two weeks Janice was
gone.

I am not a pitcher who puts on a game face, looking
as though he were about to be executed when it's
his day to pitch. If you saw me on the day of an
important outing, you'd probably think I'd pitched
yesterday. Until thirty minutes before a game, I
don't think much about what I have to do. I just
look forward to the chance to play.

Nick and I had a great trip over to Stockton,
shooting the breeze all the way. Nick is a member
of the Giants' management; his assignment was to
get me to Stockton and back, and handle the press.
From my apartment we traveled across the San
Francisco Bay and through Oakland, then up into
the dry, rounded hills of the California coast range.
Going through the Altamont Pass we viewed the
most spectacular display of windmills you'll ever
encounter—thousands upon thousands of whirl-
agigs, beating the air in symphony.

Stockton is a mid-sized farm town, the kind of
place people from the Midwest don't believe even
exists in California. A feverish afternoon breeze
was kicking up from the deep-blue sky by the time
we reached the park.

Nick and I had already heard, over the radio,
that the game was sold out. Some of the San Francisco radio stations had announced that I'd be
pitching, and urged fans to attend. From all over

northern California, Giants fans were making their way to the event.

Even knowing that, I wasn't prepared for what I found at the stadium. Hebert Park had a nice feel to it. It's part of a recreational area, surrounded by other ball fields and a picnic area. The grandstand goes up only twenty-five rows or so, with the press box squatting at the top like an afterthought. I doubt those stands were often, if ever, full. When you play A-ball, you get used to obscurity.

Today, however, fans were lining up two hours before the game. Some of them recognized me and yelled out, wishing me luck. Already, there was excitement in the air.

In all my years of pitching, I can't think that I'd ever played a game in which the fans came just to see me, apart from my team. Something different was doing here.

I began to realize that this was more than an ordinary baseball game. These fans hadn't come to yell at the umpire and cheer for home runs. They had come because my comeback was touching their hearts. They were putting their hopes on me.

The San Jose Giants had not yet arrived when I entered the clubhouse. It was a mess: cans and bottles and papers all over the place. I sat down and chatted with some fans who came by. A few minutes later the team came in from their bus, rowdy and excited, and we had a chance to get acquainted. I went around shaking hands, and finding out who would play behind me. I told the outfielders I hoped they had brought their running shoes, because I was going to pitch quickly and they might have to run after the ball quickly.

Before we went out on the field, I took time to pray. I bowed my head in front of my locker and was quiet, putting the whole game before God. I told him that I trusted him with my life, and that my intention was to glorify him in whatever I did, win or lose.

Then I went out to the playing field, and the fans went nuts. It was a standing-room-only crowd, forty-two hundred fans who seemed to want to make as much noise as forty-two thousand. The stadium wasn't big, but it was bulging. There were extra people everywhere, pressing up against the fence, straining to see, making noise.

The atmosphere called me back to my minor league days, when baseball really was a game, not a business, and there was a closeness and an excitement on the team that the major leagues don't match. This was my kind of baseball: a kid's game. I got excited.

Since the minor leagues use a designated hitter, I did not take batting practice. Fifteen minutes before the game I warmed up in the bull pen with my catcher, Danny Fernandez. I told Danny the pitches I threw, and that the backdoor slider was my "out" pitch. Danny said later that he didn't believe me. In A-ball, nobody has the control to curl a backdoor slider over the outside corner of the plate. That's why they're there: to learn control.

While I was warming up, the lineups were announced. "And on the mound, making his first appearance of the 1989 season, number forty-three, Dave Dravecky!" The announcer pronounced it with a flourish, and the fans cheered lustily. By then I was extremely nervous. It was a minor league game, but I had major league jitters.

I talked to the pitching coach, Todd Oakes, over the noise of the crowd. I told him certain keys to look for in my pitching mechanics. One was my set point. When I go into my windup, raising my arms and kicking up my leg, there's a momentary pause just before driving off my left foot toward the plate. It's very important that I be in balance then, not drifting forward or back, not going to one side or the other. I asked Todd to watch for that. I also wanted him to make sure that I had my throwing hand well above my elbow when I released the ball. That's important because it keeps me driving in a line toward the plate. If my arm drops down I tend to throw across my body, which is hard on my arm and bad for my control. And finally, I told him to watch my front foot, to make sure that I wasn't planting it stiff-legged. These were all familiar signs for Todd. He promised to watch for them.

The game began, with our guys coming up first. An outfielder named Jim Cooper, one of the Giants' young prospects, bunted his way on. Hustling all the way, he stole second, and the number three hitter singled him home. I ran out to the pitcher's mound leading 1–0.

I have a habit, when I'm going out to pitch the ninth inning, of yelling, "Everybody on their bellies!" It means, "Don't let anything through the infield! Dive for the ball!" That's what I yelled to the players before I threw my first pitch of the game.

I took my warmup pitches. The catcher threw through to second base, and the infielders whipped the ball around before tossing it to me. Then the first batter stepped in.

I toed the rubber and took a deep breath. I got the sign from Danny Fernandez. I wound up and threw. The batter swung and got a piece of it, fouling the ball back. Strike one. I threw again. Another foul, strike two. The third pitch he hit for a weak fly ball. The left fielder gathered it gently in, and I had my first out.

It felt natural. This was something I knew how to do. And it was fun. Take the ball from the catcher. Hold it and find the rubber with your foot. Look for the sign. Lift, turn and kick, throw, follow through. Lift your glove to receive the ball again. Nothing to it. Two ground ball outs later I was in the dugout, kidding around with the guys.

People told me later they had never seen someone have so much fun playing baseball. It wasn't an act. I was having fun. After I got through the jitters I was like a kid in Little League.

Every time I ran out to the mound, the fans gave me a standing ovation. There were people standing all the way down the first-base line, beyond where the stands stopped.

Because we were playing the first part of a doubleheader, the game was only seven innings. The sun was high when we began, and sank slowly toward the left-field fence, glaring straight and hot into our eyes in the visitors' dugout. We picked up another run in the second. Meanwhile I went through the first three innings without giving up a hit. My fastball was crisp, mainly in the low eighties, but topping out at eighty-eight miles per hour. My breaking pitches didn't break much, but I'd expected that. I had good control.

In the fourth inning I gave up my first hit, a single to left. That gave me a chance to use my pickoff move. My first throw over to first was a little off-target. I hadn't practiced the move, at all. I was rusty.

I looked in at Danny Fernandez, and he signaled for me to throw over to first again. I came to the set, looked at the runner—and when I made my throw, the runner was already headed for second, completely fooled. The first baseman took my throw, wheeled and fired to second base, cutting him down. That got my juices flowing!

It was a good thing we got the out, too, because the next man up hit a double, and he was followed by a batter who pounded a line drive to right. Fortunately, my right fielder caught up with it before it came down, and the inning was over.

The fifth and sixth innings went quickly, except that I was beginning to feel tired. I hadn't walked anyone, but my pitches were coming up, which is always dangerous for me. I escaped any problems until the seventh—the final inning.

The first batter up smoked a double. I got the next man on a little fly ball, but by then my arm was weary and my control going fast. I walked the next hitter, putting the tying run on base—a terrible sin.

The sun was almost down. Deep green and golden colors painted the field. I took a deep breath, and delivered to the batter.

He was bunting on the first pitch, trying to move the runners into scoring position.

He squared and made a good bunt down the third-base line—good in placement, but he had popped the ball into the air. My instincts kicked in. I took two quick, lunging steps and made an all-out, headlong dive for it, extending my mitt. I thought I could catch the ball before it hit the ground, and double off one of the runners. I got the ball—and watched it pop loose, out of my mitt.

Getting to my knees, looking to second, I grabbed the ball and pumped toward the bag. I saw that I would be late; the runner from first was already hitting the dirt. Danny Fernandez, my catcher, was beside me screaming, "Third, third!" I threw it there to force the runner from second, who had hesitated too long when I'd dived for the ball.

Out number two.

Boy, did I feel good. I wasn't a member of the walking wounded any longer. I was a pitcher, playing the only way I know how: all out, nothing held back. I'd gotten my uniform dirty.

I don't even remember how I got the last out. I just remember all the players congregating on the mound, slapping me and yelling as though we had won a playoff game. The crowd was yelling too.

The truth is, when I search through my baseball memories, I don't find any game happier than that one. I was on top of the world.

After the game I wrapped my arm in ice—one of the best sensations in baseball, to a sore-armed pitcher—and called up Al Rosen. I told him how the game had gone: seven innings, a complete-game, five-hit shutout, in which I'd thrown seventy-six pitches, reached eighty-eight miles per hour with my fastball, and only walked one. I told him I felt great. I wanted to go to Triple-A Phoenix. "Please, can I go? I want to go, Al."

He said to give it a few days, and see how I felt. He suggested that I come to talk to him in his office.

The next day, at home, I talked to him over the phone. He asked how my arm felt, and I said I had less soreness than I could ever remember. "Hey, Al, maybe now that I've only got half my deltoid muscle, I'll only get half as stiff."

"Dave," he said, "we want you to stay with the San Jose Giants instead of sending you to Phoenix. Because you know what? I don't want you diving for any balls. What do you think this is? You're going to get yourself hurt again."

I was really disappointed. I didn't say anything, but I was thinking that it would be next to impossible to keep from diving. That's the way I play.

"We don't want you to take any chances on getting hurt," Al said, "so we're going to keep you with the A-ball club for one more outing. Then, if you do well enough, we'll make the evaluation and you can go to Phoenix."

I went to Reno to pitch my next game. That meant flying on a quick hop over the Sierra Nevada Mountains, into the high desert country of western Nevada. The air is thin there, and at the ballpark the wind was blowing big time out to right field. It was not a pitcher's environment. The ball would carry to the moon.

When I got out to the mound to warm up, I found it was flat. That really brought back life in A-ball, where the groundskeeping is unpredictable and you can hear your wife's cheering in the stands.

Reno is a co-op team, meaning that they aren't part of one of the major league franchises. The players are castoffs, released by the regular teams but not yet ready to give up on baseball. Co-op players tend to be a bit wild-eyed, as you would expect given their situation. Most of them are on their way out of organized baseball. Their only hope is to play so superbly that they catch the eye of another team.

Reno's stadium was a little ratty, battered and unpainted, as though the whole operation might crumble at any time. For this game, however, it was nearly full. Once again people had heard about my comeback from cancer, and had come to see for themselves.

Maybe because of the mound, I started without good control. I immediately gave up some shots, and then a three-run home run. Some of the Reno players had been in Double-A baseball, and knew how to hit. It did not look like my night.

I made some adjustments, though, and settled down in the second and third innings, avoiding giving up more runs. My guys got some runs back, and we went into the lead.

Then in the fourth inning, as though the floodlights had suddenly switched on, it happened. I locked in. Up until then, even in Stockton, I hadn't felt it. I'd been all right. But this was different from all right. I felt I could hit a spot with my eyes closed. My breaking ball started snapping. For the last five innings I shut down the Reno team. I completed the game, throwing about one hundred pitches, and we won 7–3.

I came off the mound and told Duane Espy, the manager, "That's it, Duane. I'm ready for Phoenix."

He laughed and said, "Are you sure? I could use you around here for a few more games."

I called up Al Rosen and told him about the game. This time he said okay. I could join the Phoenix team in Tucson, and see how I did against Triple-A competition.

During the game I'd passed word around the dugout that if we won I'd take everybody out to dinner, wives and girlfriends included. The guys showered and changed in a hurry. We went to one of the casino restaurants and celebrated. Nobody had a better time than I.

The bill was truly awesome, but it was worth every penny. Minor league ballplayers don't get to live it up very often. For that one night, though, we did it right. I hope their memories of those two games are half as good as mine. They gave me something precious, and I owe them.

Pack Your Bags

I had six days of rest before I pitched in Tucson. Kelly Downs, a fellow Giants' pitcher, was already there doing rehab, and because of his pitching schedule, I had to wait a couple of extra days.

In the meantime, Janice and the kids came back from Ohio. For two solid weeks I'd been in Foster City without them, rattling around our empty apartment. The day after they returned I left again, flying into Tucson.

When I arrived at the hotel, Gayle Gardner from NBC was waiting for me. I went straight to the hotel recreation room for a long interview with her. It was another indication that my return to baseball was attracting attention. Ever since Stockton, I'd felt a growing awareness, like water piling up behind a dam.

After the interview, I grabbed a ride to Hi Corbett Field with the Phoenix manager, Gordon Mc-Kenzie. Kelly Downs was pitching, so there was no pressure on me. I had time to do some running and adjust to the Phoenix heat. After doing my work, I settled back to enjoy the game.

Kelly got hit hard that night, and lasted only a few innings. There was no reason to be surprised.

Rehabs often go that way. It served as a reminder, though, that I might be with Phoenix for some time.

The level of skill in Triple-A is not all that different from the major leagues. In addition to the regular players, I'd face Kevin Bass, the Houston Astros' slugger. He was playing with Tucson while recovering from a broken leg, and hitting .400 at the time. Kevin had always hit me hard. If I could get him out, I thought I could handle anybody.

Bob Kennedy, one of the top people in the Giants' front office (and catcher Terry Kennedy's dad), was coming in to watch me and report to Al Rosen. The Giants' pitching staff was hurting. My buddy Atlee had damaged his knee making a slide into second base; Scott Garrelts had strained a hamstring, and Rick Reuschel had a groin pull. Kelly Downs was out for an extended period of time, and Mike Krukow was done for the season. The Giants needed an arm to stay in the pennant race. The possibility of being that arm made my internal thermometer rise. I wanted to get to the big leagues, badly. I could see it. I could taste it.

Now that the end of my struggle was in sight, it was tempting to forget about living one day at a time. I could easily have zeroed in on my goal, forgetting about anything else.

That is why, before the Friday game, I took time to pray. I asked the Lord, not for success, but for clarity. I asked that he would either swing the door to the major leagues wide open, or slam it shut. I didn't want the situation ambiguous. My desire to succeed was so strong I thought I might push myself into a situation I wasn't really ready for, either physically or spiritually. I prayed that God would keep directing my path.

The way the game went, there was no doubt about which way the door was swinging. My pitching was the best yet. I didn't give up a run until the eighth inning. I didn't walk a soul. I got Kevin Bass out. (He hit the ball hard, but was one for three on the night.) And I was locked in, with the old familiar feeling.

In the eighth inning I got rocked a bit, giving up two runs. In the dugout, Gordy McKenzie asked me whether I wanted to stay in the game. We were clinging to a one-run lead.

I didn't hesitate. "This baby's mine," I told him. "I'm closing. That's all there is to it, Bud. I'm going to win or lose this game."

I must have had some fire in my eyes, because Gordy said, "Okay, it's yours. I wouldn't have it any other way."

I went out and shut them down. We won the game, 3–2. I had given up seven hits, struck out three, and walked none.

After the game I made a beeline into the clubhouse. I was looking for Bob Kennedy. I knew he'd be on the phone to Al Rosen, and I wanted to get my two cents in before he called. I couldn't see anything to be gained by more time in the minor leagues.

I spotted Gordy in the clubhouse. "Where's Bob?" I demanded. "I want to talk to him. Has he called Mr. Rosen yet?"

Gordy gestured toward the offices in back. "He's talking to him right now," he said.

So all I could do was wait. I got an ice wrap on my arm and stood around talking to some of the other players. They were fired up too. They had intensity in their eyes and their voices.

Then I saw Bob Kennedy out of the corner of my eye. I called to him.

"Mr. Kennedy! Mr. Kennedy! Did you talk to Al Rosen?"

He walked over to me slowly, a little smile playing on his face. "Yes, I talked to him. I just got off the phone."

"What did he say? Don't you think I'm ready to go up to the big leagues?"

His voice grew softer. "Well, Dave, we think you probably had better stick around at this level for a little longer. If you can get a little more work, maybe a few more games . . ."

I dropped to my knees. I knew he was messing with me. "Please, Mr. Kennedy, I'm ready. I want to go. Please send me to San Francisco."

He just looked down at me with that little smile.

"Pack your bags," he said. "Get out of here. Get your flight to San Francisco first thing tomorrow. You're going to the big leagues."

August 10

I flew back into San Francisco on Saturday morning, the day after I'd pitched in Tucson. Everything was topsy-turvy at home. Janice and the kids had stomach flu. Janice's brother Randy had just adopted a baby, and he, his wife Kim, and their two boys—counting the new baby—were staying with us while he met California adoption requirements. Our small apartment was jammed.

Yet Janice was glowing. She kept saying, "David, I just can't believe this."

Even Jonathan and Tiffany were excited. When I'd had surgery they'd cheered the news that I'd be home all the time, but as I'd slowly worked my way back, they'd picked up our feelings. Each time I'd prepared to pitch they'd asked, "Daddy, are you going to pitch in San Francisco?"

Now, I told them, I would finally be in San Francisco. Tiffany ran off cheering. "Hey, Mommy, guess what! Daddy's going to pitch in San Francisco!"

We didn't realize how many other people were getting excited. To us, my return to the majors was a miracle—*our* miracle. We knew that some fans were interested—after all, four thousand people had shown up in Stockton—but we had no idea how many.

Not until Tuesday. By then Roger Craig had named me as Thursday's starter against the Cincinnati Reds. My parents had flown in so they could see me pitch. We were driving over to their hotel room when my dad mentioned something they'd heard on the car radio.

"David," he said, "do you know anything about this Alex Vlahos thing on KNBR?"

I had to think a minute. "No," I said. "I don't think so." Alex was a little boy with leukemia whom I'd visited in June at Stanford Children's Hospital.

"You'd better listen to this," Dad said. He turned on the car radio to the station that broadcasts the Giants. Before a minute had gone by we heard my name. They wanted listeners to make a pledge for every pitch I threw in Thursday's game. The money would go to the Life-Savers Foundation, to test possible donors for bone marrow transplants of the kind Alex needed.

It's been slightly embarrassing that people have talked about the campaign for Alex as though it were my idea. All I've done, actually, is cooperate in the efforts of other people.

In June, when I was at the low point of my therapy, Pat Gallagher from the Giants' front office sent a member of his staff, Duffy Jennings, to ask me about going to see Alex. It took me about a heartbeat to say yes. I've always tried to cooperate with such efforts, but since my surgery I've become more anxious than ever to help.

COMEBACK

Certain kinds of leukemia can be cured with a bone marrow transplant, but the treatment depends on finding a perfect match with a donor. For two unrelated people, the odds are one in fifteen thousand. That means a lot of potential donors need to be tested. Alex's parents reasoned that if I visited Alex, local TV and radio stations would cover the visit and publicize the appeal for donors.

I don't enjoy the attention and publicity that come with playing major league baseball, but I recognize that once people put you up on a pedestal you can't take yourself down. You have a responsibility to act wisely and generously in the role you've been given. I don't agree with players who feel they don't owe anything to anybody. Everything I have is a gift from God, and I am responsible to use it accordingly.

So I gladly went down to see Alex. We met on a big lawn in front of the hospital. It's a lovely spot, with a sense of luxurious space you don't often find at a big university hospital. Stanford was founded on Senator Leland Stanford's old horse ranch one hundred years ago, and there's still plenty of open turf shaded by huge oak trees.

Alex, who was six, was an incredible bundle of energy. The TV cameras and reporters were there, but Alex wasn't awed. Nor was he awed by me. He told me he's a big Giants fan, and he especially looked up to Will Clark and Kevin Mitchell. Fortunately I had brought him one of Kevin Mitchell's bats.

Alex was completely bald from all the treatment he'd been receiving, but otherwise he was a normal kid. We played catch, and I pitched a few to him so he could hit with his Whiffleball bat. At one point, when I was talking to one of the reporters about my desire to glorify God, Alex looked at me and said, "You love God a lot, don't you, Dave?"

I said, "I sure do, Alex."

"I do too," Alex said. "I love Jesus." That was really neat for me, because I got a chance to encourage him to keep putting his faith right there.

We spent an hour and a half together. Since that day I'd tried to keep in touch with Alex and his parents, and I had sent Alex some small Giants mementos. But as far as I was concerned, the publicity was done.

As matters developed, publicity had barely begun. Every time I got into the car and turned on the radio, they were talking about me and the game I would pitch. On Wednesday, Janice got out the little portable radio she always keeps in her purse, and we listened to the radio on and off all day. By Wednesday night I knew something much bigger than Dave Dravecky was happening. They had not stopped talking about me all day. I was the news in San Francisco. Period.

I tried to explain it to Atlee. He was in Birmingham, Alabama, having a knee operation.

"Atlee," I said, "it's incredible. I mean, people are acting like this is the biggest event in history." I told him about the campaign for Alex. By game time the pledge was over $1,000 per pitch.

Atlee was trying to fool the doctors into thinking that he had recovered enough to fly home and see the game. "I don't think they were fooled, Dave," he said. "The doctors said there is no way they are going to let me out of here."

I told him it didn't matter. "Don't worry about me," I said. "I'm just going to go out and do my best, and whatever happens, happens."

But I was fired up. The night before the game I told Janice there was no way I would sleep. I was just too excited.

When my head hit the pillow, though, I must have been out in ten seconds. I slept so soundly Janice had to wake me up in the morning. Since it was a day game, I needed to pick up Scott Garrelts by 9:00 A.M. I was still sleeping at 8:30, and had to hustle into the shower.

Before I left, we had a brief family prayer. All week we'd had tremendous commotion in the house, with guests and friends coming and going, but that morning we had a few quiet moments alone before I left. We were upstairs in our bedroom, Janice and I sitting on the edge of the bed, Tiffany and Jonathan standing next to us. We all held hands and said some very simple prayers.

We prayed for my peace of mind. We really had no idea how the game would go. Even when I'd had all the muscles in my arm, on any given day I could go out to pitch and get shelled. So we prayed that whatever came, I'd have a sense of peace and calmness, and that I'd be able to glorify God through the way I performed. We didn't pray that I'd win—we never do that—but just that my attitude and my focus would be correct.

And we gave thanks. We thanked God that he'd brought us to this point.

Janice began crying. Suddenly in that quiet moment she realized what we were doing. Until then she'd been moving too fast.

Her tears upset Jonathan. "Mommy," he said, "what's wrong?"

Janice was too choked up to answer him.

He turned to me. "Daddy, why is Mommy crying?"

"Jonathan," I said, "those are tears of joy, not tears of sadness, because Daddy's going to pitch again. We never dreamed that this day would be possible. And here we are."

I picked up Scott Garrelts in our Volvo station wagon. Scotty is a quiet, lanky, slow-talking guy from the farm belt, somebody who doesn't make speeches. But he'd worked his way up to giving one that Thursday morning. He'd figured he had to give me a pep talk.

I spoiled it for him, though. I had a tape playing on the car stereo, and it was blasting so loud that Scott wondered if he'd need some cotton for his ears. The tape had a song that I especially like, "Give Thanks with a Grateful Heart." When that came on I really cranked it up. Scott decided his speech was unnecessary.

Thanks is what I felt. I'm never a psycho about pitching. I don't work myself into a fit on game day. But August 10 I felt especially lighthearted and almost eerily relaxed. My heart was full of thanks—thanks to God that I had the opportunity to pitch again, to do what I love so much. I was excited, but not worried. Win or lose, I was living a miracle. The doctors had told me that I would never pitch again, and today I was going to pitch.

COMEBACK

The clubhouse was quiet, a kind of refuge from the turbulence of the outside world. I got dressed and went out on the field to take batting practice. The day was overcast and cool. Many summer days in San Francisco start out with a high overcast that burns off by the afternoon, but that Thursday the weather stayed put, hazy and gray.

I followed my normal pregame routine, going back into the clubhouse to take it easy. I try never to focus on the opposing team until about thirty minutes before the game. I just try to relax, as if it were any other day.

I went into the training room and lay down on one of the tables, just to shoot the breeze with the trainers or the players there. I lifted some light barbells, going through a few quick sets. I took a look at the *San Francisco Chronicle*. My name was all over the front page.

When it was close to game time, Brett Butler and Bob Knepper, two of our veteran players, came over to my locker and said they'd like to pray. We asked Mark Letendre, our trainer, whether we could use his room for a few minutes of privacy. Scott Garrelts and Mackie Shilstone, the strength coach, joined us. They prayed with me for about ten minutes.

Then I went back to my locker and put on my white game uniform. "Giants" was blazoned across my chest, and "43" across my back. It looked good. It felt good. I glanced into my locker and saw the two balls that Norm Sherry puts there for each pitcher on the day he starts.

*   *   *

Fifteen minutes before the game, I walked down the runway, a dimly lit concrete tunnel. Reaching the door that opened onto the field, I stepped into the glare of a brightly overcast day. For a second I was disoriented. In a long, ragged row in front of me, along the entire sixty-foot length of the bull pen, were photographers and TV cameramen pointing their lenses at me. The cameras were whirring like a battery of machine guns. I looked at Norm, the pitching coach, who was standing by the door. "Holy smokes, Norm, what is going on?"

He just smiled. By then I probably could not have heard his answer, for the crowd had caught sight of me.

The San Francisco bull pen is set along the first-base foul line, in front of the right field grandstand, exposed to everything. The fans were yelling like crazy. I began taking off my jacket, and the cheering continued. It seemed to spread, up and out through the whole ballpark.

I just wanted to start throwing the ball, as quickly as possible. I strode to the mound. But by the time I got there, the whole, huge stadium— 34,810 fans—were on their feet, giving me my first and undoubtedly my last ever standing ovation in the bull pen.

Terry Kennedy was my catcher. During the winter the Giants had traded for him, and at the time Janice and I had talked about—just dreaming— how wonderfully appropriate it would be to have Terry catch me if I came back. He'd been my receiver when I broke into the major leagues, and he's a guy I like and respect tremendously. He also knows my pitching better than anyone.

My heart was racing, a hundred miles an hour. The noise was incredible. I looked at Terry and grabbed a bit of jersey over my heart, pounding it up and down to show him how my pulse was hammering. I pointed at him: "You too?" TK looked back and, with a big smile, signaled that his heart was doing the same thing.

Then I began to throw, just playing catch with Terry. As soon as I made the first toss, a sense of peace blanketed me. All I had to do now was what I know how to do best: throw a baseball.

I warmed up quickly, as I always do. In fact, my arm got warm faster than I wanted, and I had to stop for a while so I didn't wear out before the game. It's possible to leave your best fastball in the bull pen.

When I was ready I walked down to the dugout. The cheers followed me. People were standing again. I could hear them yelling crazily in the stands, "Go get 'em, Dave!" "We're glad you're back, Dave!" In the dugout the guys were fired up.

When it was time to go out on the field, I yelled, "On your bellies!" I jogged out to the mound and heard the crowd noise grow, swelling to a roar. They were standing, cheering for me. The score-board in center field flashed a gigantic, "WELCOME BACK, DAVE."

I stood holding the ball, rubbing it, looking at Terry Kennedy. I jerked off my cap and waved it in acknowledgment of the cheering. I couldn't pitch. I was suddenly overcome with emotion—with all the built-up emotion of the past ten months of struggle. I looked around me, up and up at the rows upon rows of cheering people, rising around me so that those at the top looked like bright-colored dots. I have no words to describe my emotions. My heart was full.

I stepped off the mound to gather myself together. I thought, *Now is as good a time as any, before this all starts, to say thank you, Lord. Just thanks. Thank you for the privilege of doing this again. Thank you that you restored my arm so I could pitch. But most of all, thank you for what you've done for me. Thank you for saving me. Thank you for your love in Jesus Christ.*

It didn't take long to do that, just a few moments. Then I stepped back up on the mound and started throwing. Immediately I was locked in. My rhythm and balance came effortlessly. From the first batter, Terry Kennedy and I were thinking together on pitch selection. It was just a picture: Terry and me playing catch, as though nobody else was around.

I had the kind of stuff that makes the other team look like they're not trying. As I've said, I'm not a pitcher to blow people away. I move the ball around, hit spots, catch batters leaning the wrong way, bust their bats with an inside pitch. I'm a pitcher who frustrates batters, because they're so sure they'll get me, until—What do you know!—they've gone 0 for 4.

The first one or two innings are the most important to me. Once I get in a groove, I can sail.

The Cincinnati Reds were certainly not conceding the game out of sympathy. However they might have been touched by my comeback, they were touched more by the fact that we were in a pennant race. On August 10 we were in first place by two games. The Reds had been picked by many to take the division. They wanted to beat us. That's what the game is all about.

One of the sports writers had asked Pete Rose, the Cincinnati manager, whether he'd thought about the enormity of what I was attempting. Pete spit out a sunflower seed. "No," he said bluntly. "He's back, and it's great for him. I hope he loses."

The first hitter was Luis Quinones, the Reds' hustling second baseman. I started him off with a pitch high and outside, ball one. That set up the fastball inside. He turned on it, hard, and smashed the ball down the third-base line. But he had pulled it foul.

I thought he would be looking for that inside pitch again, so I went low and outside with my backdoor slider, and picked up a strike. The count was one and two—much to my advantage. That's the way I like to pitch. Throw strikes, get ahead of the batter, and make every pitch a pitch of purpose.

The purpose of the next pitch was to get him swinging at a bad pitch. With two strikes he was vulnerable. But he laid off a slider outside.

I came back with the same pitch, only closer to the plate. I just missed the outside corner, and he took it for a ball. I think the call could have gone either way.

I now had a full count. I'd gone outside with three straight pitches. So I went there again. I thought he might still be thinking of that inside pitch he'd fouled off. I put my backdoor slider on the outside corner of the plate, just slicing a piece off the very edge. He had to dive down to get it, and all he could do was loop his bat and pop a fly ball into center field.

One out. The cheers rained down.

The second batter went quickly. I started him out with a fastball inside, and then came back with another which he grounded right at Matt Williams at third base.

Eric Davis was the third man in their lineup, one of the toughest hitters in baseball. I went outside with him. With Eric, anything inside is likely to end up as a souvenir.

But I missed with my first two sliders outside. Behind in the count, I needed a strike. If in doubt about what to do, keep the ball down. I threw a sinking fastball over the plate. Davis hit the ball solidly, but on the ground. Matt Williams, with those wonderfully gentle hands of his, gobbled it up and threw across the diamond for an easy out.

As I ran in to the dugout, the crowd stood for another standing ovation.

That's how it went through seven innings. Every time I trotted in from the mound, the crowd stood to cheer. Janice, watching in the stands, cried continuously for two hours. It's a good thing that Tiffany and Jonathan were perfectly behaved; if they had been in any trouble, she might not have noticed.

Alex Vlahos was there. His mother said he hadn't been eating much, or wanting to play with his toys, for the past two weeks. But when he'd heard I would be pitching, he'd told her that peanuts sounded good to him. His mom offered to get some from the hospital cafeteria. "No, Mom," he'd said, "I mean the kind they sell at the game." He'd come to cheer for me.

Roger Craig said later that in all the decades he'd played and coached, he'd never seen so much emotion at a game. It was half revival, half baseball game.

I had near-perfect control. Only four times did I go to three balls on a batter. I walked only one, toward the end of the game. And I entered the eighth inning having given up only one hit, to Joel Youngblood in the second inning. I made up for that by popping him up the next time he batted, and striking him out the third time.

In the meantime, my guys were giving me the support I needed. In the second inning Pat Sheridan laced a ball into the left field corner, racing all the way around to third while Joel Youngblood chased it down. Terry Kennedy came up next and hit a ground ball to second, good enough to score our first run.

Then, in the third inning, Will Clark connected with an outside pitch and drove it opposite field, down the left field line for a one-out double. Kevin Mitchell followed Will. Since Kevin was the major league's leading home-run hitter, Pete Rose elected to walk him. The strategy was foiled by Matt Williams, who nailed a pitch to straight-away center field. Eric Davis dived for it, but couldn't come up with the catch, and a run scored. With runners on second and third and only one out, we failed to score more. But we were up 2–0.

It became 4–0 in the fifth. Kevin Mitchell walked again, and Matt Williams made the Reds pay again by crushing a first-pitch fastball into the left field seats.

It turned out that I needed those runs.

In the seventh I began having some control problems. The ball began coming up. I didn't give up a hit, but I had to throw a lot of pitches.

Nobody particularly noticed. When you go into the eighth having given up only one hit, the manager is not thinking about pulling you.

I started off the eighth inning by breaking Todd Benzinger's bat. Unfortunately, the ball looped off his fists over Robby Thompson's head for a single. One of those little things again: a fluke hit, and most dangerously, a leadoff hit.

Oliver, their catcher, was next. My first pitch to him was out over the plate, a pitch he might have hit a mile, but he didn't have a good swing at it. He hit a routine fly ball to left field. One out.

Their rookie third baseman, Scott Madison, came up next. I threw exactly the same pitch I'd thrown to Oliver, and Madison killed it. It bounced off the wall in left, and he coasted in with a double.

With men at second and third and just one out, Pete Rose pinch-hit Ron Oester for Rob Dibble, their pitcher. Oester gave me a tough at-bat. We battled to a three-and-two count. And then I punched him out. He swung and missed a backdoor slider. The crowd roared. I pumped my fist.

Two outs. One more and I was out of trouble. Luis Quinones was up. The count went to two balls and one strike when I threw him my bread-and-butter pitch, a backdoor slider. It wasn't a terrible pitch. It was up a little. It didn't break much. Quinones, who is no big slugger, turned on the ball and got all of his bat on it. The little white pill sailed high and deep to left, and I watched it with a sinking heart. It went over the chain-link fence in left field, suddenly a souvenir for the kids who scramble after balls.

I felt sick for a minute. One bad pitch, and a four-run lead was reduced to one. How quickly the game can change.

It had happened so quickly that Roger didn't even have a pitcher warming up. I went ahead and pitched to their shortstop, Richardson, who grounded weakly to short.

Going in to the dugout, I got another standing ovation.

I knew I was done. I was due to hit in the bottom of the eighth, and despite my great hitting that day—I'd walked twice—I was sure Roger would pull me. Sure enough, Kirt Manwaring went out to hit for me. Roger called on Steve Bedrosian, our stopper, to pull the game out of the fire.

I wasn't going to take a shower with my game on the line. I stayed in the dugout. I wanted to see "Bedrock" get the final outs.

When Bedrosian went to the mound to warm up, the crowd started yelling. It took me a minute to realize that they were cheering for me. They wouldn't stop.

Terry Kennedy was next to me. TK yelled, over the din, "Go on out there. It's your day. Take a bow." He nudged me. "C'mon, get going."

So I did. I went out on the field, looked up again at those rows upon rows of fans, yelling their lungs out, and I lifted my cap. It was my twelfth standing ovation of the day.

I went back in the dugout, but the fans wouldn't stop. It was as though they had a need to cheer, a need to pound their hands together and let out some of the emotion. They wanted me again. Some of the guys were gesturing at me. "Go out again! C'mon, Dave!" I walked up the steps. I looked up again at the thousands upon thousands of people whom I would never know, but who shared that moment with me. I lifted both my hands to the fans, in thanks.

Bedrock was full of fire. He threw heat, and the heart of the Reds lineup couldn't handle it. Eric Davis grounded to short. Herm Winningham struck out. Ken Griffey struck out. Like that, the game was over.

I was on my feet before the last swinging strike. Terry Kennedy grabbed me for a hug. I ran out toward the mound. Other teammates were grabbing me, slapping me on the back, congratulating me on the game. Will Clark was one of the last to reach me. He opened his arms for a great big embrace. The fans were still cheering, yelling as though they'd never stop, even as I walked off the field.

Janice hadn't seen the last outs. The security people at Candlestick Park had told her that they wanted to get her out of the stadium as soon as I had finished pitching. So she and the kids began wading their way slowly through the crowds, heading toward the clubhouse while Bedrock finished it off for me. Her face was a mess: red and tear-streaked. She counted the cheers, knowing that each one was an out. One. Two. Three.

The security guards led her to the long, wide tunnel where the bull pen guys come in from the game. Guys in uniforms started piling down it, headed for the clubhouse. Suddenly our rookie relief pitcher, Jeff Brantley, saw her. He's a short, stocky guy, full of bubbles. He got a big, manic grin on his face. "Hey, Baby!" he shouted. "We did it!" He grabbed her and started jumping up and down. Then Craig Lefferts, another reliever, spotted her, and *he* started jumping up and down. They were all three in a bundle, their arms around each other. Janice was sobbing.

"What are you doing here?" Jeff finally asked. Wives and family members usually wait in the players' parking lot after a game.

"I'm waiting for David," she said.

"Well, he won't come this way. Come on down to the clubhouse."

Janice had never been in the clubhouse, in all our years. The only women who come in are reporters. She was embarrassed, but the guys were excited about taking her to me.

She saw me. I saw her. I was in front of my locker, still in my uniform. Janice came over with her arms out. "Oh, David," she said.

I held her close. I looked around at the room. It was absolutely quiet. The men were just standing back, by their lockers, watching us. Afterwards they came over to Janice, one by one, and hugged her.

*　　　*　　　*

I got ice wrapped on my arm, and Janice and I went to the press conference that had been called in the 49ers' locker room. It was hard to muscle our way in. The *Sporting News* was there. *Sports Illustrated* was there. *People* magazine was there. The "Today" show was there. "Entertainment Tonight," the *Christian Science Monitor,* "CBS Morning News"—everybody who was anybody in the world of news and entertainment was there.

Roger Craig was talking. He'd told them how emotional the game had been for him, and how he thought its importance had reached far beyond baseball, sending a message to people all over the nation who face sickness or difficulty. Then Roger handed the microphone over to me.

It was quiet in the room, almost as though no one quite knew where to start. I took a question. But I realized, almost as soon as I began answering, that I had something I needed to say for myself, before I forgot it in the rush of questions.

"Before I take any more questions," I said, "it's important for me to give credit where credit is due. I want to give praise and glory to Jesus Christ for allowing me the opportunity to come back and play again." I went on to credit my doctors, my therapists, and my trainers, and all the others who had made it possible. But I tried to make clear that in my mind, my comeback was a miracle for which God deserved the praise.

The press conference went on for a long time. There were often long, quiet pauses between questions. I believe the reporters were still trying to absorb what they had seen and heard.

Many questions had to do with my future. How

did I feel? What did I anticipate about the rest of the baseball season? I told the reporters that I hoped to be able to pitch normally from that time on. "I feel great," I said. As to the future, I would have to take that one day at a time. "But after what happened today, anything else is icing on the cake."

Janice and I finally got away from the ballpark, loading up a van and a carful of our visiting relatives just in time to get stuck in phenomenal traffic. We listened to the radio. The game was the only subject, no matter what station you tuned to, even on national news. It was as though God had allowed the whole world to take a day off, just to focus on our little game in Candlestick Park.

We went to dinner with my parents and some family friends. Afterwards, Janice and I decided to drop by Atlee and Jenny Hammaker's home. We pulled into the parking lot at the same moment that they arrived from the airport. Atlee had just come in from Alabama, too late for the game. He'd heard the score, but he wanted to know details. We talked until midnight.

When we got home at last, there were twenty-six messages on our answering machine. Friends from everywhere we'd ever lived were calling. Plants and flowers had been arriving all day, and more were on our doorstep and at the neighbors. The place soon looked like a greenhouse.

Then, finally, it was time to go to bed.

Janice and I were alone for the first time since the morning. We knelt beside the bed to pray, as we often do—me on my side, Janice on hers. For a moment there was quiet. Then I lifted my head and I looked over at Janice.

"Have you taken in what happened today?" I asked. "Have you absorbed it yet?"

"No," she said. She gave a big sigh. "No, I haven't, David. It's like I'm a spectator."

"Me too," I said.

The Pitch

THEN, suddenly, everything was normal. For the previous ten months—or longer, if you count my year of shoulder problems—I had lived with uncertainty. Would I come back? Or would I not?

After that wonderful day of August 10, the doubt was gone. Like a big wave on a Hawaiian beach, the attention had grown, surged, lifted us, pulled us along—and then run on to something else, leaving us in the calm, bubbly water of its wake.

We began to realize that we could live a normal life.

It felt oh, so good to go to the ballpark that weekend and work out as a regular team member, as a player who was making a contribution beyond cheerleading. It even felt good to wake up Friday morning with a pitcher's normal next-day stiffness—to flex my arm and test it, to notice the soreness in my leg from kicking and in my hip from rotating, to feel the muscles in my back and chest. In the clubhouse, I was just one of the guys, not a special case any longer. No matter how many times they'd told me I was one of them, it hadn't really been true—until now.

On Sunday the team had no batting practice, so

The Pitch

Janice and I were able to go to church together—a pretty rare treat for us during the regular season. My mom and dad were staying on for a while, so we spent our spare moments with them. And we basked in the glow of what had happened.

I was particularly excited by some of the letters that the campaign for Alex Vlahos had generated. For example, two letters came from the Sonoma Development Center, a state facility for the mentally disabled. One was from a member of the professional staff, explaining that David and Harry were two elderly men who have spent their lives at the center. For fifty years they've been a team. Harry can't speak, so David talks for him. David can't walk, so Harry pushes his wheelchair. They're avid Giants fans, who listen to every game. When they heard about the campaign for Alex they went around with a jar and collected $29.62 in my honor.

The second letter was from David and Harry themselves. They wrote:

Dear Mr. Dravecky,

We are donating money to the little boy that has leukemia. Harry and I put money pitch by pitch in our fund. You went eight innings and we were proud of you.

People helped us out so we want to help someone else.

Sincerely,
David and Harry

I sent them a signed baseball as a thank-you.

I later heard that it was their most prized possession.

There were other letters addressed to the radio station:

The enclosed check is not to honor a pledge. It is in memory of our six-year-old grandniece who died last year because they could not get her a bone marrow transplant.

It is a wonderful thing which you have done to assist Dave Dravecky in calling attention to the need and filling it.

God bless you all
I. and B. M.

Gentlemen:

Please accept the enclosed $100 check as my contribution toward Life-Savers. I was lucky enough to have been at the 'Stick this afternoon and I'm still feeling blown away by the experience. The fact that Dave Dravecky was able to pitch so well after having gone through what he's gone through was amazing in and of itself; but I find I'm even more impressed by the strength of character and inner serenity that he's exhibited throughout his ordeal. He's one of the only people I can think of whom I would describe as truly inspirational, and I feel honored to be able to donate some money in his name toward a cause that he considers worthwhile. I wish I could give a million dollars instead of a hundred.

This hasn't been a great year for role models in baseball, but Dave Dravecky is a happy exception to that rule. I feel proud to be a Giants fan.

Very truly yours,
S. P.

Dear KNBR staff:

I want to thank KNBR for accepting money on behalf of Dave Dravecky, and for the integrity with which you are covering his story. You have allowed him to be who he is, to speak about his faith, even though people who do not understand the impact of a genuine faith might scoff or complain about hearing his words.

Who would parents want their son to be like? I certainly know the answer for myself. It is too bad that we make heroes of people who are not heroic in their personal living. No matter how much we may like some of Elvis's music, the world will survive without any of it. It will survive without baseball, and I am a loyal, enthusiastic Giants fan! It will not survive without the moral integrity and faith integrated into life as exhibited by Dave Dravecky. Dave is not perfect, I'm sure; no one on earth is. But he is an inspiration to us all, a true example of a great person, whose life multiplied many times would make our country a far safer and a more caring and rewarding place to live!

Appreciatively,
S. G.

COMEBACK

Dear KNBR,

I don't believe in miracles, but I was at Candlestick yesterday when Dave Dravecky and the Giants beat the Reds. I do believe that certain individuals because of their faith, dedication, or perseverance, can create a rare moment in which thousands of people experience a genuine unselfish feeling of brotherhood. A feeling which transcends race, religion, prejudice, and yes, which even transcends baseball at a Giants game.

Dave Dravecky is one of those inspirational individuals.

He inspired me to do several things I don't normally do. I don't usually write letters or send money to radio stations, and I don't usually think kindly of my fellow human beings, in general. So as a result of that tremendous day yesterday at the Stick, I'm sending $50 in Dave Dravecky's name to the KNBR Care Fund, for Alex and all of the other kids like him.

Sincerely,
M. B.

There were many, many more letters. I don't know how these affect you, but they touched Janice and me very deeply. It was an incredible feeling to sense that we were being lifted up and above our own workaday concerns, that our lives were being used to encourage and help and challenge others whom we did not even know. Clearly, it wasn't our doing. All we'd thought about was making a comeback in baseball, doing it the best way we could, always trying to keep our focus on God's will, not our own. God had taken that and made much more of it than we could have imagined.

We had a very strong sense that, though our lives were returning to normal, "normal" would never be quite the same again. We had seen what God could make out of "normal." "Normal" was an adventure.

It was apparent that people had heard what I'd said at the news conference about the credit belonging to Jesus Christ. One of the *San Francisco Chronicle* reporters, in fact, wrote a column about the issue a few days later. He described his mixed feelings about the "God Squad" of Christian players on the Giants, and his inner conflicts in reporting my press conference after the game. He said that he'd gone up to the press box and found many writers huddling together, asking, "Are you going to write about God?" or "How much God are you going to put in your story?" He admitted that he'd chosen not to mention God when he wrote his report. Among other factors, he was afraid of turning people off.

I can identify with that. I've often felt intimidated, knowing that some people weren't going to like hearing me talk about my faith. But I'd decided that, in as nice a way as I could, without being pushy, I wanted to say what I truly believed. In the day-to-day reporting of baseball, God isn't a big factor. Christians don't pitch very differently from non-Christians. But it just wasn't possible to talk about my comeback without naming Jesus Christ. Without him, there would have been no story to tell. Part of the satisfaction that came for Janice and me, in the backwash of that incredible day, was our sense that I'd had the opportunity to take a little bit of the spotlight off Dave Dravecky and turn it toward God—for to him the glory truly belonged.

On Monday I left with the team for Montreal. For once, I was really excited to hit the road. For a year I hadn't traveled with the team, excepting the two trips I'd had in June and July with my family along. After all the activity I'd been through, I looked forward to the less complicated life of traveling with my buddies, playing ball.

It's a long, weary flight back east, and going into Montreal takes you through customs, so I didn't get to bed until late. But that was okay. When I'm on the road I keep California time, staying up until 2:00 A.M. on the East Coast, and getting up late the next morning. Tuesday's game was at night, so I'd have all day to relax. I was due to pitch.

The next morning Bob Knepper and I got together and headed out toward a bookstore Bob wanted to visit. The day was overcast and cool, but it was good to be out walking the downtown streets. Montreal is a beautiful city, and I like to be active on the day I pitch. If you lie around the hotel, you may find yourself with a tendency to lie around at the ballpark. You feel tired because you've been feeling tired all day.

Bob had joined the Giants the same Saturday I'd flown in from Tucson. He'd been released by the Houston Astros, and the Giants had picked him up to strengthen the pitching corp. I knew Bob slightly. He had a reputation for being very strong-minded, which made some people shy away from him, but I like strong-minded people, being one myself. I also love books, and Bob, I knew, read every book he could lay his hands on. I thought it would be neat to go to a bookstore with him.

Walking along, we got talking about my experiences of the past week. I told Bob about the thankfulness that had filled Janice's and my hearts, and how wonderful it felt to be back on the team.

"Bob," I said, "you just have no idea how exciting it's been to live in the middle of a miracle. There I was on the mound, putting the ball where I wanted it, getting guys out. It was unbelievable. Then besides that, to have a press conference jammed with reporters, and get a chance to give the credit to Jesus Christ. Of everything I've done in baseball, that's the top."

We'd been talking about that for a few minutes when Bob threw a new idea at me. "Dave, it's great that you've had a chance to give God credit for your comeback. But I see another miracle that transcends what's happened to your arm. That's the miracle that God began in your life eight years ago in Amarillo. It seems to me that's where we ought to place our focus. It's great that God's given you another chance to pitch. But that's pretty small, compared to the chance he's given you to live life with him eternally."

I don't think Bob had thought through what he was saying until the words came out of his mouth. It really hit us both, simultaneously. Bob wasn't correcting me, he was just bringing out the larger picture of what was going on.

"See, the way I understand it," Bob went on, "we can talk about our experiences all we want, and it's good to give God the glory when we are able to overcome obstacles. But let's face it, we live in a lost and dying world, and people need to know more than that God helped you come back from cancer in your arm. They need to know how Christ can begin to transform their lives, just as he's transforming yours. They need to know how they can break down the barriers between themselves and God. In fact, they need to know that those barriers have already been broken down by what Jesus did for them on the cross."

We continued on our walk, on to the bookstore and then to lunch. All the way, as we walked, we kept discussing the perspective Bob was bringing. It took me some time to fully grasp what he meant, but when I did, I felt deeply excited and challenged. What, after all, did my comeback mean to people? What good did it do to encourage and inspire them to try harder, when they weren't sure why they were alive?

Under the roof of Montreal's domed stadium there were perhaps twenty thousand fans that night, a good crowd but nothing extraordinary. They gave me no standing ovation. I wasn't looking for one. I was looking for a chance to win my second game of the season. I was back to normal, and this was a normal game. That's the way I wanted it.

After three innings, I felt confident. I'd gone through their batting order without giving up a hit. When I came to bat, I *got* a hit myself. I wasn't throwing quite as hard as I had five days before, and my control wasn't as sharp, but I was moving the ball around, keeping it down, and making the adjustments that were necessary to win.

In the fifth inning I struggled with my control, but Roger Craig wasn't thinking about warming up a relief pitcher. He thought I was cruising along. After five innings, I'd given up only three hits and no runs.

In the dugout after the fifth, I was rubbing my left arm. It felt strange. It didn't hurt, exactly; there was a tingling sensation.

Brett Butler, our center fielder, was standing near me. He noticed what I was doing and came over. "Is everything all right?" he asked.

"Yeah, everything's fine," I said. "I just feel a little stiffness." The tingling felt as though it came from my muscles.

Long ago, Dr. Muschler had warned me that if I ever felt any pain in my arm I should quit throwing immediately. He'd warned me about the possibility of a fracture. But I wasn't thinking about that. I'd done so much in the months since those warnings, and I'd never had the slightest problem. The thought that this was a warning sign never crossed my mind.

We made a little excitement at the plate in that inning. Will Clark singled, and with one out Matt Williams tagged one deep. That made the score 3–0 when I jogged out to the mound for the bottom of the sixth. The heart of the Expos lineup was coming up.

I started wrong, coming out over the plate to Damaso Garcia and watching the ball fly over the left field fence for a home run. Andres Galarraga was next up. I came inside, just as he was diving out over the plate expecting an outside pitch. I'd fooled him, but the pitch was too far inside. It nicked him. He went down to first base.

Robby Thompson came over from second. "You feeling okay?" he asked.

"I feel great!"

Three thousand miles away in California, Janice was sitting by the pool at our condominium complex, talking with my mom and dad and watching Tiffany and Jonathan swim. The game wasn't on TV, so she was listening on her little portable radio. When I hit Galarraga she got nervous, just like a manager, because my control wasn't good. She began talking to Roger Craig. "Get him out of there, Roger," she said. "Take him out before he gets into trouble." Roger wasn't listening.

Tim Raines came up. I had the ball in my glove, and I rubbed it thoroughly. I was unhappy about putting a runner on base, and I knew I would have to bear down to get Raines out. He's a very tough hitter, and he represented the tying run.

I came to the set position, stared over at Galarraga at first, then pivoted on my left leg, at the same moment pulling my left hand up and back for the pitch. Pushing off the rubber, I threw.

Next to my ear I heard a loud popping noise. The sound was audible all over the field. It sounded as though someone had snapped a heavy tree branch.

I felt as though my arm had separated from my body and was sailing off toward home plate. I grabbed at my arm instinctively, trying to pull it back. The ball left my hand and flew high up, far past an astonished Terry Kennedy, who went charging after it.

But I knew nothing about the ball, or about the runner who ran hesitantly around the bases, as though, for once, he was truly guilty of stealing. I was grabbing my arm to keep it from flying away, and tumbling headfirst down the mound. I shouted with all the air in my lungs. Over I went, doing a complete 360-degree tumble, then flopping forward until I came to rest on my back, my feet pointing toward center field. My arm felt as though I'd been hit with a meat axe. I have never felt such pain. I wish that no one else ever would.

In an instant Will Clark was there, looking down at me. I was writhing and grunting, trying to get my breath. "Oh, gosh, Will, it hurts, it's killing me! It's broke. It's broke. It feels like I've broken my arm."

Changing My Focus

EVEN through the pain, my thoughts flowed vividly and clearly. As I fell, grabbing my arm, I found that my arm was still attached. When I hit the ground I thought that the bone must have punctured my skin and be protruding out of my shoulder. I didn't want to touch it, but I had to find out. Carefully working my right hand up my arm, I found that everything was intact.

A muscle must have torn loose, I thought, or the shoulder dislocated. But moving the shoulder around, I could tell that wasn't so. The pain came from elsewhere. I made my instant diagnosis: I must have broken my arm.

These thoughts whizzed through my mind in a matter of seconds. Meanwhile I was shaking and grunting and crying out from the pain. My skin had broken into a heavy sweat. Above and around me, the stadium had fallen awesomely silent. You could have heard somebody eating peanuts in the upper deck.

Mark Letendre, our trainer, was beside me in a flash. Because of the pain, I was holding my breath for long periods. Mark started to tell me how to breathe. "In at the nose and out at the mouth,

Dave! In at the nose! Now out at the mouth! C'mon, Dave, breathe with me!" He was giving me a Lamaze refresher course.

I gasped, between breaths, "I'm all right. It just hurts."

"Shut up, Dave, and breathe. In at the nose . . ."

The pain gradually subsided until I could lie quietly, looking up at the circle of faces. Roger Craig, feeling helpless, leaned down and hugged me. Mark was checking my arm.

Meanwhile, apart from the tumult around me, even apart from the pain, I was thinking another set of thoughts. I was simply amazed at what was going on. I'd thought the book had been written on my comeback, and I could go back to normal. Now this.

I wasn't, not even for a split second, angry. I was simply astonished, and full of the certainty that God was writing another chapter in my life. Something more, something amazing, was being revealed.

They brought a stretcher next to me, and wanted to get me on it. I said no. "Let me walk off," I said between gritted teeth. "I'm all right."

"Shut up, Dave. You're not walking."

I didn't want to go off the field horizontal. I'm not that kind of guy. So I asked if I could at least sit up. They reluctantly said okay. The stretcher had an aluminum frame that could be positioned for that.

Getting onto the stretcher was no picnic, though. As soon as I started to get up, I realized that my left arm was just hanging. When I moved, the pain shot through it and seemed to take over every nerve in my body. I didn't want anybody touching it. I finally managed to struggle into a sitting position, and onto the stretcher. They wheeled me off, through the tunnel and into the training room. There they put me on a table.

Scotty Garrelts was standing near me, with tears in his eyes. "Dave, do you want me to call Janice?" he asked.

I said yes, call Janice.

"What do you want me to tell her?" Scott asked.

"Tell her I'm all right. Tell her I think I broke my arm."

She was listening to the game by our pool, and didn't at first realize how seriously hurt I was. The radio announcers deliberately down-played my fall; they didn't want to frighten people by describing what they had seen. Janice was more worried about Andres Galarraga going on to third than she was about me.

There was a long pause in the action. Janice heard one of the announcers say he couldn't really see what was happening because I was surrounded by players from the Giants and the Montreal Expos. She stood up, realizing that something was seriously wrong. She grabbed her radio, wanting to make it say more, wanting to get inside it so she could see. She almost threw it. Tears began streaming down her face.

She ran into the house, leaving the children to my parents, and called the Hammakers. Jenny answered the phone. She said that Atlee (he was home recuperating from his knee operation) would call Montreal and try to reach the clubhouse. Janice hung up and waited, pacing, listening to the radio. A few minutes later the phone rang. It was Scott. He told her what I'd said.

For the rest of the evening our house was in chaos—the phone ringing, people coming over, the kids running in and out, and Janice waiting to hear more news.

In the clubhouse, Dr. Brodrick, the Montreal Expos' medical director, appeared. He was trying to get me to move my arm into another position. I finally told him it just wouldn't work; my arm hurt too much. So he and Mark Letendre taped me up. They wrapped my arm tightly against my body, as though I had it in a sling.

A handful of players and coaches were watching while the doctor did his work. Al Rosen, the general manager of the Giants, stood there, looking stunned. So did Bob Knepper.

Ballplayers are not big on showing emotion—not emotion of the tenderer kinds, at least. That day, though, emotional currents were rushing out of control. Terry Kennedy expressed the feelings well when he told a reporter, "I've known Dave a long time, and he's probably as good a friend as I've got. As hard as he's worked to come back, this is not supposed to happen to people like him. This is not supposed to happen to good people."

After the game, Roger Craig was completely unable to speak. He broke into tears in front of reporters, who had to wait in embarrassed silence for a solid minute before he could talk.

But the game continued while I lay in the training room, and only a handful of players were present. Suddenly Mike Fitzgerald, the Expos' catcher, came running in with all his catcher's gear on. Danny Gausepohl, whom I'd played with in Amarillo, is Mike's uncle. Through Danny, Mike and I had become friends.

Mike looked at me with tears in his eyes, grabbed me by the back of my head, and pulled me next to him. He hugged me and kissed me. "I love you, brother," he said, and turned and went running out. I just watched him go in amazement. I'm fairly sure *that* had never happened in baseball before.

An ambulance arrived, and they were about to wheel me away when Bob Knepper put his head near mine and suggested that we pray. I looked at Al Rosen and asked whether that would be okay. He said to go ahead. Brett Butler had come in, and he put his hand on me. Bob had a hand on my shoulder.

I don't remember what Bob said. I'm sure he prayed that peace would descend on me. It wasn't what he said, though, so much as how he said it. Bob had a hard time getting his words out. His voice was cracking, and he had to speak slowly to get his words through. Love for me permeated his prayer.

While he prayed, the inning had ended, and Giants' players came racing in from the playing field. We could hear them running toward us, and then, as they entered the room, falling silent. By the time Bob finished, the room was jammed with twenty-five guys, all dead silent. There was an overwhelming sense of emotion. I looked up and saw that many of my teammates had tears in their eyes.

For me, Bob's prayer took away any remaining anxiety. I knew I was in God's hands.

As I was being wheeled out, I turned to Terry Kennedy. He was standing next to me, his eyes full of tears, staring as if to say, *What on earth is going to happen to you next?*

"Hey," I said, "if there was ever anything to the old cliche 'Win one for me,' this is it, guys. I don't want that lead to evaporate, because I'm probably not going to pitch again this season, and I want my record to be 2–0. I want to end the year undefeated."

Terry looked at me as though I had lost my mind.

Then I greeted the ambulance driver. "This has been kind of a rough day," I told him, "so please get me there safely. I've had enough excitement already."

What do you do in hospital emergency rooms? Wait, of course. They wheeled my stretcher into a hallway and I waited while Giants' officials signed forms and answered questions. I got somebody to call Janice and let her know I was okay. Eventually I was taken in for x-rays, and the doctor who had seen me at the ballpark came down and examined me. They determined that I had a broken arm, a clean fracture with no other damage apparent. It was while I was at the hospital that I first began to speculate that the break might be a result of my bone being frozen.

After the doctors put on a cast, they saw no reason to keep me at the hospital. Somebody called a taxi and, shortly before midnight, I headed back to my room. I was anxious to get to the hotel. I wanted to be with my friends.

I hadn't taken any pain pills, so I was squirming with pain. But my frame of mind was almost bizarre, it was so positive. I'm no masochist, and I certainly didn't enjoy breaking my arm, nor would I care to ever repeat that falling-off-the-mound trick. But emotionally I was still riding the excitement that had begun on August 10, and had been kicked up a notch by my talk with Bob Knepper. I felt a tremendous sense of thankfulness and expectancy. I had no idea what was going to come next on this adventure, but I trusted that God had wonderfully good things in store for me. I could almost see him cutting away the thickets, and my destination becoming clear.

When I got back to the hotel room, still in my uniform, I called Janice. Mostly I wanted her to hear it from me that I was all right.

I was propped up with pillows, sitting on my bed. A few of my teammates were starting to drift down to my room as the word spread that I was back. They came in slow and serious, as if they were at a funeral, but they soon realized that it wasn't that kind of atmosphere. I was so glad to be with those guys.

Scott Garrelts was there, and so was Jeff Brantley, who had come in to relieve me when I'd broken my arm. I'd heard at the hospital that we'd won the game. While I was talking to Janice, I saw Steve Bedrosian out in the hallway. Bedrock had come on in the ninth once again to preserve the game; we'd won by another one-run score, 3–2.

"Hey Bedrock! Bedrock! Way to go! Thanks for saving the game, man! Now I'm 2–0, and I've got some negotiating power for next year!"

I was feeling pretty rowdy for someone who's just broken his arm. Janice said it sounded like a party was going on.

Pretty soon it settled down to me, Scott Garrelts, Jeff Brantley, Greg Litton, and Bob Knepper. We raided the mini-bar in the room, drinking up all the Cokes and eating all the chocolate bars. I was starting to feel really hungry, so we sent Jeff and Scott out for some fast food. They were gone for about an hour, and came in soaking wet and carrying a ton of junk food. They'd been running all over Montreal in the rain, trying to find a hamburger place, and had finally ended up catching a taxi which took them to Burger King.

By then it was probably 2:00 A.M. I knew it was going to be tough for me to sleep, since the doctors had commanded that I sleep sitting up.

"Hey, why don't we just stay up all night?" I suggested. If I was going to be awake I wanted company, and we were having fun.

We stayed up until 5:00 A.M. We discussed our marriages, and the importance of putting our wives first in our schedules. We talked baseball. We talked about the pressures of competition. We laughed a lot. And I shared what Bob and I had talked about that morning. Under the circumstances, the truth of his remarks was more evident than ever.

When there was light leaking over the horizon, we closed our time together with prayer, and the others disappeared to catch some sleep. I felt a wonderful sense of peace. I took some Tylenol with codeine, and managed to doze for two and a half hours before it was time to get up again.

At about 8:00 Scotty came down to my room and stuck his head sheepishly in my door. "Hey, Dave. You said I should come down."

"Yeah. Come on in."

I was still wearing the same dirt I'd picked up falling off the mound. My hair was filthy. I'd asked Scott to help me get ready for my trip. In particular, I'd asked him to help me wash my hair. I didn't think I could manage it with my cast on.

I really don't know who was more embarrassed, Scotty or me. It was a pretty ridiculous scene: two grown men, reputed to be athletes, trying to get one man's hair washed. I will spare you the details. It did feel great to get clean. Scott helped me pack my gear and get ready for the trip.

The Giants' management had asked whether I'd mind holding a small press conference before I left, just for the beat writers who cover our games. I'd said sure.

The press had been summoned to a small hotel suite. Fifteen or twenty reporters were circled around with their tape recorders or notebooks.

Bob Knepper and Scott Garrelts stood in the doorway, listening and praying for me. I began with a simple statement, telling the reporters the same thing that I'd been talking about and thinking about constantly for the past twenty-four hours.

I told them that the real miracle in my life had nothing to do with an operation on my arm. It had to do with something Jesus Christ had done for me two thousand years before, when he had died for me and made it possible for me to live in fellowship with him. I just said it as simply as I could, and then I took questions.

With my arm breaking, the focus had shifted. The press had written about my comeback as a miracle, but what could they call this? The opposite of a miracle? If coming back from cancer had lifted people's hopes, should this dash them? That wasn't how I saw it. I saw my life as one continuous adventure in partnership with God. The miracle of my life had begun in Amarillo, and it continued.

I told the writers that I hoped to be able to come back and pitch again. I had no intention of quitting. But that wasn't the basic source of my optimism. My optimism was grounded in Jesus Christ, and that day, particularly, my emotions were flooded with thankfulness for what he'd done for me.

For the press, too, the focus had shifted. Before, they had told the world about my physical recovery. Now they reported on my attitude, as if that were more mysterious and awe-inspiring than my arm.

It was a long flight home. At the Montreal airport there were reporters, and in Chicago there were reporters, and when at last I reached San Francisco there were reporters by what seemed to be the hundreds.

Janice had been brought up onto the walkway to the plane. I could see the worry in her eyes, and imagine how difficult it must have been for her to wait for me. We had a few moments to kiss and greet each other.

Security police were everywhere. They led me out past the gate to a podium. People cheered as I emerged. The room was jammed; even the balcony overlooking us was jammed. I felt like the President of the United States.

I was starting to drag with fatigue, but I tried to answer all the reporters' questions. Then we were led downstairs to the runway, where a limousine was waiting. It took us to Palo Alto, where I had x-rays taken and confronted the press again. Then we went home.

Tiffany and Jonathan were glad to see me, but they were awed by the limo. They decided that I was more important than they had thought.

We went to the Hammakers' for dinner. My mom and dad were there, rather quiet. We sat in the living room for a few minutes, and I told them what the day had been like. Then Jenny called us in for a tremendous lasagna dinner.

I sat at the table, looking around me—at my wife and kids, my parents, my best friend and his family—and I felt very, very grateful to be alive.

I was extremely tired. I felt as though I'd lived a lifetime in a day.

Tomorrow I would have a lot to consider. I didn't know what my future in baseball might be. But whether I pitched again or not, the right response was still the one I'd blasted Scott with on the way to the game just six days before: Give thanks. Give thanks to God with a grateful heart.

A Second Comeback?

ON August 10, I would have thought that media attention had reached an absolute peak. Surely no more attention could be showered on Dave Dravecky.

I soon found there was another level. On August 15 all the late news programs began their coverage with the horrifying film of my arm breaking. Soon every major network wanted a special interview. Dozens of magazines and newspapers were calling. So was Hollywood, to talk about motion pictures.

I was not anxious for the attention. I was in considerable pain from the break, and I was getting little sleep propped up in a sitting position. My life was chaotic enough. However, within the limits of my time and my stamina, I tried to talk about what I had been through, and how I understood its meaning. I invariably included some words about my faith, since I could only understand what had happened to me within that context.

Janice and I began to receive a flood of mail. Though we tried, we couldn't answer it all. But it affected us deeply.

We were driving down the freeway together, on

our way to see Dr. Campbell, when I read aloud this letter:

Dear Dave,

God bless you! You're the type of guy I always thought I'd be. I really do care, and I'm a loving person, but I've made a tragic mistake, and I'm now at San Quentin's death row. I was an idiot and got involved in cocaine, and it has cost me my life as well as the life I took.

I have written the warden twice to see if there's any way we as Christians here can try to help Alex Vlahos. If they could get even one third of the inmates at Quentin and Folsom, his chances of getting the proper donor would really increase. I know Alex is not the only one with that sickness, so if they gave us the tests and kept records, we could possibly help others.

It's really hard being a Christian here because there is so much hate. But we do hold Bible studies and fellowship with one another.

I just wanted to say get well soon. I actually cried when you fell off the mound. I know it took a lot to come back. You can imagine what my life is worth here. Everyone thinks we should all be killed, and even though the real me didn't take that life, I deserve to die. You may think I'm crazy, but if there's any way to transplant a new bone in your arm, you can have mine. I'm truly serious. I'd be honored. I would just like to help any who are in need.

I'm making a card for Alex before I send this, so if you could give it to him when you see him, and give him a hug for me, please tell him there's a lot of brothers here praying for him.

And Dave, if you want the bone it's yours. Like the news said, you'll be prone to fractures. Mine has never been broken.

Love in Christ,

J.

P.S. You can have my muscle, too, if it will help.

When I read that to Janice I got about halfway through and had to stop. I was amazed that such a man could offer me such a gift.

Another letter came from a mother whose son attended the same school as my daughter Tiffany. She wrote:

Dear Dave and Janice,

I am a single parent and my son has not seen his dad in four years. In February he started Little League here in Foster City. From that first practice he loved the game.

Dave, when you shared at school my little boy was like a sponge absorbing every word you spoke. The main reason for this note is to say thanks. I know this has been a year of peaks and valleys. In your joys and pain you've given our Lord the glory and you have helped teach my son what a godly man is.

I too have had tough trials in my Christian walk, but God's grace is sufficient. Please know you are in our prayers. I know you must have many people in your life, pulling in all directions. I just wanted to thank you for making a difference in my son's little life. Thanks too for making your life an open window so little boys all over this country can see Jesus in a man they admire and respect.

In Him,
K. H.

And then there was this note from a friend who had played professional baseball some years before:

Dave,
I could not find a card that said, "Sorry your arm broke, but I am praising the Lord it did!" I, like many others, pictured you pitching the winning game of the World Series, but our great God had a much bigger and better plan. You became a household word when tragedy struck, but in that you had the opportunity to tell the whole world of your faith in God. God knew you would do that, that's why he ordained the comeback. I prayed every day for you, so I was not at all surprised when all of our prayers were answered. I am excited for what the Lord has in store for you and your family. I will continue to pray daily for you.

In his great love,
L

Many, many other letters came, some from those who shared our faith and some from those who didn't, but all from people evidently touched by something they'd observed in watching me or reading about me. Janice would sit with a stack of this mail, reading snatches to me, dabbing at her eyes with a Kleenex. It's an awe-inspiring experience to discover that your lives have been affecting people whom you've never met.

Breaking my arm had not put a stop to that. Rather, it had drawn even more people toward us.

That made sense, when we thought about it. Not all obstacles can be overcome. Each of us needs grace to handle troubles that remain even after we have done everything we can. A prison inmate needs grace to come to terms with his past, which he can't erase. A single mother needs grace to raise her son without a father. Some barriers cannot be broken down just by human effort and faith in yourself.

When my arm broke, people who didn't even care about baseball reached out to us. They identified with the heartache. They were inspired, I believe, by my attitude in response. Some wanted to know the secret. Where did I get the ability to respond positively, without bitterness?

I wasn't the only person getting press coverage. Both Dr. Muschler and Dr. Campbell held press conferences to explain what had happened to me. Dr. Muschler later told me he was embarrassed to become a celebrity just because his patient had broken his arm. They'd tried to guess how long it would take me to recover fully from the surgery, but there had been no track record on which to base their guesses. Obviously, they'd guessed wrong.

The break was what Dr. Campbell called a spiral oblique fracture, a break that is common in skiers' legs. My humerus bone must have been weak, still recovering from being frozen, and the tremendous, repeated stress of pitching had opened a hairline crack, a stress fracture such as basketball players often suffer in their feet. The tingling I had felt before the sixth inning had probably been from such a fracture. If I had remembered Dr. Muschler's warning, if I had stopped and taken myself out of the game, he would have ordered me to take two weeks off, and I could have been pitching again in six, just in time for the postseason. *If*.

As it was, the prognosis did not sound too awful. Nobody had ever pitched after losing his deltoid muscle, but plenty of people had pitched after breaking an arm. Dr. Campbell said that I was done throwing for 1989, but he saw no reason why I couldn't return in 1990. Fortunately, the broken bone had done no damage to muscles or connective tissues. The break should mend stronger than ever.

I was back in uniform when the Giants returned home on August 25, ten days after my arm broke. The guys were curious about whether I would stick around with the ball club. I told them that I would definitely stay. I was determined to be at every practice, to be in uniform cheering at every game. I wanted very much to be a part of the team.

My teammates were appreciative of my support, and there was some talk about how I served as an inspiration to the team. But the truth is, we were in a pennant race, and we had to win games with good pitching, good fielding, and good hitting—not inspiration.

Before, when I'd been on the bench, I'd had the hope of eventually playing. Now I was watching, showing up for practice, cheering from the bench, but without any possibility of eventually making a contribution. All I could do was to stand around. I couldn't even ride the stationary bike, with my arm in a brace.

I wanted to be out there, especially as we entered late September and our first-place lead dwindled to just a few games. The San Diego Padres were on our tail, and just wouldn't quit winning. It was hard for me to watch, and not play.

It was during that period that I heard from my agent, Jerry Kapstein. He said that he'd approached the Giants about a contract for 1990, but the ball club didn't seem interested. Al Rosen, our general manager, wanted to talk to me personally, Jerry said.

Janice and I had a long, heartfelt conversation that night. Was the door closing on my career in baseball? If the Giants weren't interested in keeping me, there wouldn't be a lot of other teams waiting for a chance to sign me up. Janice and I firmly believed that if one door closed, it was because God had something else in store for us. We began praying that we'd recognize a new door when God opened it. Still, I carried a sad feeling in my heart for about a week. The team evidently had considered their options and decided against me.

I finally got to talk to Al Rosen. He asked me up

to his office, and I walked in expecting to get the bad news from him personally. Al is a trim, handsome, silver-haired gentleman, a former All-Star third baseman. I have tremendous respect for him, not only for his knowledge of baseball, but for the way he does his business. He's honest. And he truly cares about his players. It was no accident that he'd been in the training room in Montreal, after I broke my arm.

When we got through the small talk, Al told me that he wanted to offer me a contract for the following year. I was floored. I walked out of that office feeling great. For some reason, the Giants had reversed their evaluation of my potential. I never found out why, and I probably never will. I was just happy to know that the team still wanted me, and the door was still open for baseball.

We finally clinched our division title in the last week of the season, while we were in Los Angeles. I'd asked for permission to travel with the team because I wanted to be there for the celebration.

We lost to the Dodgers—in fact we got swept—and had to wait in the clubhouse while the San Diego Padres went into extra innings with the Cincinnati Reds. If the Padres won, we would have a showdown at their home park.

All the lockers had been covered with plastic to protect clothes from the champagne we were expected to shoot at each other. TV cameras and reporters were jammed in with us. In a back room, where they keep the bats, somebody had a radio, and we would occasionally hear a cheer or a groan go up from there.

A Second Comeback?

Finally, the word spread with a shout: the Padres had lost, and we had clinched the division title. I was standing near Al Rosen, and we hugged each other. Then I went through the clubhouse, laughing and slapping and hugging my teammates. Even though we'd lost that day, there was no shortage of excitement. Through six months of play, we had played the best baseball in our division. That's what you work for and hope for every season: to come out on top. You rarely achieve it. Now we had to prepare for the Chicago Cubs, who had won the National League's eastern division.

The Playoffs

NOT everybody was pleased at my response to a broken arm. Most of the sports reporters downplayed my faith. A few took public exception to it.

A writer for the Palo Alto *Times Tribune,* for example, devoted a column to me, headlined, "This kind of preaching doesn't have a place in the sports pages." He wrote, "People say they're tired of reading about million-dollar contracts, about colleges that cheat, about drug scandals, about athletes who beat up women in bars, and all the other repugnant aspects of life that are interwoven into athletics.

"Well, I have a complaint as a reader and viewer, too. I'm tired of reading about God in the sports section. . . ."

I thought that was a remarkable comparison: putting God on the same level as drug scandals, cheating, and beating up women in bars.

But the writer, Chuck Hildebrand, went on to make remarks that many people would agree with. "Religion is, or should be, a private matter and an individual commitment. I don't discuss my religious beliefs with most people, mainly because they aren't anyone else's business, and I think it's rude to impose beliefs on anybody else. To make a public spectacle of religious feelings only cheapens them."

He suggested I was shortchanging myself by giving God credit. "God didn't lift those weights and endure those excruciating exercises and overcome the fear that his career might be over. Dravecky did."

His message to me, if I wanted to talk about my faith: "Go buy air time or take out an advertisement, Dave."

Though I don't agree with him, I know he was speaking for many. "Religion is a private matter," some people say, by which they apparently mean, "Don't mention it in public." If a reporter asked me the secret of my perseverance, apparently I should blush and respond, "That is a private matter which I never discuss with anyone but my wife and my psychiatrist."

I never want to push my beliefs on anybody. There's a time to talk about Jesus Christ, and a time that's inappropriate. When a reporter asks me what pitch I threw to a certain batter, I don't bring God into it. He asks the question expecting a factual answer, and I give it to him.

I don't think it's quite fair, though, for a reporter to insist that I censor the true story of my comeback. Certainly God didn't lift any weights for me, but he did give me the courage and the perspective to deal with adversity—and even with heartbreak. If some find that distasteful, there are others who truly want to understand what makes me tick.

For some people, religion is so private they never want to talk about it. That's their privilege. But does that mean they should impose their version of religion on me? Faith makes a visible, demonstrable difference in my life. It permeates my thinking and my behavior. If I stop talking about it, I'd have to stop talking about practically everything important to me.

Still, I sometimes needed wisdom to know when to talk, and what to say. I received many opportunities to speak, sometimes for large amounts of money. Some I reluctantly declined, because the context wasn't right for saying what I believed, and I didn't want to watch my words. At any rate, I couldn't possibly do even a small proportion of all I was asked to do.

As the letters and requests kept coming, a burden of helplessness grew. Janice and I knew we couldn't speak everywhere. We knew that we could never respond to the many questions people raised in their letters. Even if we had been free to do nothing else, we would not have been able to answer them all personally. That's when the idea of writing a book began to grab us.

Along with the many reporters, producers, and agents who had contacted us were a number of publishers. At first we had grouped their offers with all the others. We began, however, to think that a book might offer an opportunity to share ourselves. We could tell our story in our own way, using our own words, to those who were truly interested.

We began meeting publishers. At first it was exciting. We met some people we genuinely liked, who seemed to share our vision. But then, gradually, the excitement turned to weariness, and we felt we were in an even greater quagmire.

The weeks around the 1989 playoffs were extremely difficult for Janice and me, more difficult than anything we'd encountered after my surgery. Even when I'd been banged up from the operation, even when I'd hit the wall in rehab, we'd really never lost hope or encouragement. Now, though, we struggled. Janice does not normally cry much, but she cried more than she had during our entire married life.

One factor was her father's death, which came unexpectedly in September. Janice had watched him go through some great emotional struggles after her mother's death. When he died, all her sad memories, as well as the happy ones, came back.

But more of her tears probably came from dealing with me. As time went on I became more and more difficult to live with.

First off, I couldn't get a decent night's sleep. Because of my arm, I wasn't allowed to sleep lying down. We eventually rented a reclining chair, just so I could sleep propped up in a sitting position. For me, though, there is nothing like the horizontal. Night after night I tossed uncomfortably and didn't really sleep. Day after day I grew more tired.

Another galling factor was that Janice had to bathe me. I just don't like the feeling of helplessness.

And then, frustration kept building over baseball. I couldn't play. I would go to the ballpark and try to be a good cheerleader, but soon I felt like an invisible man. I wasn't looking for attention. I just wanted to be out there between the lines. In my whole life, I had never had to sit in the dugout and watch my team playing for a championship.

When I am frustrated or angry, I tend to hold it in. I quit communicating with anybody; I fall into a mood that nobody can break. Even Janice can't penetrate. Then, finally, the mood breaks out like a pent-up volcano, and I can become terribly angry. I've never hit anybody, but I've thrown things and hurt people with my tongue. Nobody sees this except my family, but it's an ugly side of my personality that I hate to even admit.

That is perhaps the area of my life that has changed most dramatically since I became a Christian. It had been years since I had fallen into that kind of mood. But when we began the playoffs, I was feeling it in me, welling up, threatening to break out.

Part of it was the book. I'd found it impossible to make a neat, easy decision about publishers. A lot of different people—people I liked and respected—were calling me up and visiting me and writing me letters, trying to get me to see the decision the way they did. I wasn't in good condition for that.

Then my teammates got involved. Atlee Hammaker and Bob Knepper, two guys I like and respect as much as anybody on this planet, took up the issue as though it were their own, and they offered very strong opinions on what way I ought to go.

I don't think anybody realized fully how I was

feeling except Janice. She knew, of course. She was watching me slip into my own moody world. She knew how little I was sleeping, too. Most of all she knew how much I ached to be on that field playing baseball.

The playoffs began in Chicago. It's one of my favorite cities to visit, and like everybody else who has ever been there, I like Wrigley Field. We had the dubious distinction of playing the first night games in its (slight) postseason history. In the first game, my guys put on a hitting clinic. Will Clark clubbed two home runs, the second a fourth-inning grand slam that put the game out of reach. We won 11–3.

Everybody was happy but me. That night I didn't sleep. I ached. It wasn't just my arm that ached, either. It was my whole body, aching to be in the game.

During the game, the television cameras were focused on me during a long exchange between Vin Scully and Tom Seaver. Seaver said my comeback was probably the most emotional story in baseball that year. Scully said, "I still marvel at how he accepted the frustration, the pain, the disappointment, and put it all in the right perspective."

At that point in time, unknown to them, I was having a hard time keeping that perspective.

The next day the Cubbies turned the tables on us. Rick Reuschel, our quiet, thoughtful veteran pitcher, got pounded for six runs in the first inning. We never caught up, and lost 9–5.

But I didn't see the end of the game.

Before the game, Bob Knepper had taken me

aside and given me a big talk about how he saw my choice of publishers. Bob is a person with strong principles, which I appreciate, but it was as though he couldn't stop selling his principles to me. He had to make his points one more time. At least, that's how I felt. At another time I wouldn't have been troubled by it. By then, though, I was not a happy camper.

Throughout the game I had that on my mind. And more, I had on my mind the helpless frustration of watching our team get beat. I wanted to play.

After the sixth inning, Atlee came up to me in the dugout. He had been in the bull pen, and had come down to share his thoughts with me.

"Hey," he said, "I've been thinking some more about the book."

"Save your breath," I told him. "I've already heard an earful and I don't need any more."

"Who gave you the earful?" he asked.

"I talked to Bob," I said.

"Well, I've been thinking about it, and there are some things I need to tell you," Atlee said. He started in with his thoughts.

My blood pressure was rising. "I don't want to hear it," I said, beginning to turn away.

"That's a great attitude," Atlee said. "Just walk away."

"Yeah, that's the attitude right now," I said. "I'm getting out of here, because I can't take this any more."

I left him, and stomped out of the dugout and upstairs to the clubhouse, where I took a shower. All the frustrations of being with the team but not playing, of feeling conflict with my friends, of lack of sleep, of uncertainty about the future—these had all reached the surface. I couldn't take any more.

When the game was over Atlee came up to me in the clubhouse and apologized. "David, I am so sorry," he said. "I know I was wrong. Can you forgive me?"

"You don't have to apologize," I said. "It was nothing. I just need my space."

"Will you wait for me?" Atlee asked. He was going to take a shower, and he wanted to walk out with me.

So I waited, and we walked out into the cold Chicago night together. I wasn't over my mood. I wanted to be over it, but I couldn't shake it.

Janice was waiting for me outside, under the stands. She took one look at my face and knew that I was unhappy. She asked me what was the trouble, and when I didn't answer she thought I was upset with her. She took it all wrong.

There were people surrounding us, meeting each other, or waiting for the bus back to the hotel. It was no place to talk.

"Janice, let's just get on the bus," I said.

We rode in silence. I felt terribly guilty for taking it out on Janice. I could foresee a whole new batch of crying coming on.

I thank God that he's helped me, over the past years, not to live under such moods, as I once did. I thank God that I've learned how to control them and escape them.

Janice is one key. More and more, I've learned

to talk with her, to share with her what I am feeling. On the plane home from Chicago, I was finally able to open up with her and explain what I was going through. I was able to tell her that I love her, that I wasn't angry with her, and I was terribly sorry that I was taking out my frustrations on her.

"I'm tired, Janice," I said. "I'm tired of people telling me what to do. I've heard it all. I just want to make my own decision."

"Well, David, if you feel that way, you should go and talk to them. Tell them what you're feeling."

Strange how a simple and obvious thing like that can be overlooked when you're in a mood.

When we got back to San Francisco I collared Bob and Atlee individually in the clubhouse.

"I appreciate everything that you've done," I told them. "I know you've been giving me advice because you love me and you care for me. But now I want my space. I want to be able to make this decision with Janice and feel comfortable about it. I don't need any more input."

They honored that request, and it half killed them, because for a long time they didn't know what I was deciding. After that, though, we could be friends again. And they are both wonderful friends.

If you only looked at the final scores of the 1989 National League championships you might think they were lacking in drama. After going back to San Francisco tied at one game apiece, we took the next two games. One more win and we had put the Cubs away.

But you'd need the whole dictionary to describe

these games. In each one, we came from behind to win, on power hitting by Kevin Mitchell, Matt Williams, Robby Thompson, and above all, Will Clark. Will put on a hitting display that has never been matched in a playoff series.

He was not the only guy hitting, though. On the other side, Ryne Sandberg was hitting with power, and Mark Grace, the Cubs' tall, slender first baseman, was rapping out line drives with every pitch in his reach. It was, as one sportswriter put it, as though the difficulty of hitting had been abolished.

We came to the fifth game determined not to lose, not to let the games go back to Wrigley Field. For one thing, we all hated the thought of another plane trip. We wanted to stay home, and since the Oakland A's had already won the American League championships, we'd be done traveling if we could just win this game.

We also had the memory of what the Cardinals had done to us in the last two games of the '87 playoffs. You can never predict what might happen in Wrigley Field, where the fences are near and the fans so close they seem to be watching over your shoulder.

The guys were extremely loose in the clubhouse before the game, laughing and joking with each other, playing cards. And yet they had fire in their eyes. Atlee suggested I get my camera, so we could have some group photos to remember the day by. When I got onto the field with a camera around my neck, Terry Kennedy jumped all over me. "Hey, get the press out of here! The press isn't allowed out here to take pictures!" It was that kind of mood.

Then, after the national anthem, the mood

changed. Suddenly the intensity hit us all, and we began screaming and yelling, pounding each other. The fans were generating an incredible amount of noise. You couldn't hear yourself.

Right from the first inning, the game had the tightness and the tension of a pitcher's duel. It was Mike Bielecki pitching for the Cubs against our Rick Reuschel. The Cubs had eaten Rick for breakfast in the second game of the series, but today he had them crossed up in every direction. And Mike Bielecki was locked in. None of us could figure out his pattern. You would be looking for a fastball outside and he would throw a curve inside. Or you'd be looking for the curve and he would break off a split-finger fastball. Will Clark came into the dugout after a failed at-bat, shaking his head and saying that Bielecki was throwing one of the best split fingers he'd seen all season.

I watched like a pitcher, calling each pitch. When our team was in the field I'd grab a seat on the bench, but when we came to bat I would squat on a bucket down at the end of the bench near the bats. I screamed my lungs out.

I really like to watch Big Daddy Reuschel pitch, because of his phenomenal control and his ability to change speeds with his pitches. I was calling each pitch for him. "C'mon, Big Daddy, bust him inside. Fastball inside!" Then he'd throw the slider on the outside of the plate and strike the batter out, and I'd think, *Great call, Dave.*

Reuschel's philosophy is to throw as few pitches as possible. He says that when a scouting report tells us a guy is a first-ball fastball hitter, ninety-five percent of the time we're warned not to give the guy anything to hit on the first pitch. But Big Daddy's philosophy is to throw him a fastball and let him hit it. Reuschel says that if he could face a whole team of first-ball fastball hitters, he could throw just twenty-seven pitches in a game—one for each out. He'd just have to throw it in a place that the guy couldn't hit it well.

We came to the bottom of the eighth inning tied at one run apiece. Bielecki had pitched almost flawlessly, giving up only three hits—one a triple to Will Clark that had allowed us to tie the game. With two outs, Roger Craig sent in Candy Maldonado to hit for Reuschel.

I'd talked to Candy before the game. While everyone else was laughing and kidding around, he had been scrunched down in front of his locker, looking miserable. Roger wasn't starting him. Candy hated to sit on the bench.

Over the All-Star break, while he was home in Puerto Rico, Candy had committed himself to follow Christ. His wife had been a Christian for a long time, and Candy had flirted with Christianity for as long as I could remember, but he hadn't wanted to give up his lifestyle. Over the break, though, through some dramatic events, he'd finally come to a point of decision.

For the first two weeks after that, he'd hit the ball all over the lot. He'd been jubilant, attributing his hitting to God. Those of us who were Christians hadn't wanted to discourage him, but we'd warned him that it didn't work that way. Jesus Christ isn't in the business of turning people into hitters.

And sure enough, after that Candy slumped to

his worst year ever in the major leagues. I have to hand it to him, though: He hung in there. He didn't quit the faith, and he didn't quit trying to play.

When I saw him in the clubhouse he looked at me with his big brown eyes full of pain and said, "Dave, I know how I'm supposed to act on the outside. I know I'm supposed to keep my feelings under control. But inside I am hurting so bad. Inside I am so . . ." He broke it off. He couldn't talk.

I was feeling some similar feelings. "Candy," I said, "I know you can't just push it aside. I know it hurts, and that's the way it has to be. But keep your focus on the Lord, and when you get an opportunity, you'll be ready."

When Candy was sent in to pinch-hit, I began to pray for him. By then I had moved off my bucket and was out in front of the bench, in my catcher's stance, screaming through every pitch. I told God, "I know you don't want me to pray like this, but I'm going to anyway, because this guy has been in a pit and I want him to succeed." I prayed that Candy would hit a home run and be a hero. All through his at-bat I prayed for him.

Candy didn't hit a home run. He did something more unusual: He showed patience. He kept fouling off pitches, working Bielecki deeper into the count. Finally he took a walk.

A little thing. A walk, with nobody on base, with two outs. But it set in motion a train of events.

Bielecki lost his game plan. He said later that he was tired, but you really should be able to throw strikes even when you are tired. Candy had pushed him to the limits and drawn a walk, and now, with sixty-two thousand fans on their feet

and their screaming wall of sound bouncing off the
concrete bleachers, each strike must have become
harder to find. He's a young pitcher and I'm sure
his heart was hammering. I know mine would have
been. He walked Brett Butler. Then he walked
Robby Thompson. And that set the stage for guess
who: Will Clark.

There is nobody I would rather have at the plate
when crunch time comes. When the game is on the
line, Will's round, dark, glittering eyes seem to
stare through you. All he sees is the baseball.

The Cubs' manager, Don Zimmer, brought in
Mitch Williams to pitch. It was the perfect
matchup: youth vs. youth, lefty vs. lefty, strength
vs. strength, our best vs. their best. Williams has
a feverish, whirling, herky-jerky delivery, and he's
often scarily wild. His nickname is Wild Thing.

I thought he would walk home a run. But his first
pitch was a strike. I knew then it was going to be
a battle. Wild Thing was throwing heat.

I also saw something in Will. He was staying in.
Sometimes he, like all lefties facing another lefty,
tends to bail out. After all, the ball comes at you
like it's heading straight for your head. It's natural
to duck, especially with Mitch Williams throwing
wild stuff that could literally kill you. But Will
wasn't flinching.

On the second pitch, a fastball, he swung but
was behind, and fouled it weakly away. He took
a ball, then fouled off a slider. He foul-tipped a
fastball high in the strike zone, just staying alive.
He took a fastball away, evening the count at 2–2.
Then Mitch threw a fastball high in the zone again,
a pitch that Will often misses, and Will swung,

locking his hips and connecting with that sweet, compact upward arc, and the ball darted, as though on an unexpected journey to freedom, cleanly over second base and into center field. Two runs came home, and the air of Candlestick was thick with sound. I swear you could have cut it and sold it by the pound.

After we went ahead 3–1, I walked back to the clubhouse to put the brace on my arm. I wanted to celebrate, and I wanted to avoid hurting my arm while I did it. I couldn't believe it: my second World Series in five years.

The fun was not over, however. As though the curse had suddenly been removed from their bats, the Cubs began the top of the ninth like batting practice, zinging hard line drives in every direction. A run came home, and the stands fell silent. I kept thinking of the 1984 playoffs between the Padres and the Cubs, when by the ninth inning people had been carrying smelling salts up and down the bench, because guys were about to pass out from exhaustion after screaming for so long. My voice was shot from shouting, and my body weak from cheering.

There were two men on and two outs when Ryne Sandberg, Chicago's great, steady second baseman, came to the plate. Sandberg is a pure fastball hitter. Steve Bedrosian was in, throwing nothing but fastballs, and getting tagged.

Terry Kennedy went out to talk to Steve. He told him to go with his slider, since the fastball wasn't working. Bedrosian's slider hadn't been very effective of late.

The Playoffs

He threw a slider, down and away. Sandberg swung and hit a soft ground ball to Robby Thompson at second. Robby wheeled and threw the ball to first. It was over. We were on our way to the World Series.

Everybody piled out of the dugout, toward the mound, jumping on top of Bedrosian and Clark, piling together into one pulsating, moving lump with legs. I followed cautiously, wanting to be careful of my arm, but wanting badly to join the celebration. I got to the pile and leaned against it carefully, watching to make sure I didn't get jolted. But I never thought about being hit from behind. Someone—I have no idea who—slammed into me. I was thrown into the pile, and astounding pain blazed through my arm. It hurt as much as it had in Montreal, though the sensation was different.

I went down into a crouch, holding the arm against my body, trying to protect it from the surging, leaping pile of bodies around me. Then Dusty Baker, our hitting coach, saw me and came to help. He and Mark Letendre pulled me out of the scrum and led me off the field, holding my arm in pain, while the rest of the team continued to celebrate.

23

Earthquake

JANICE saw me from the stands when I was led off holding my arm. From her angle she couldn't see my face, though, so she wasn't sure whether I'd been hurt. My mom and dad, sitting in another section, had seen clearly. They told her that something was wrong.

Janice went quickly to the area of fenced-off asphalt outside the clubhouse, where family members and friends wait after the game. Players, whooping and slapping hands, were coming out to hug their wives and girlfriends. None of them seemed to know I'd been hurt, and they were busy with their own concerns. Fans were crowding against the fences, looking down at Janice from above, shouting in victory celebration, and wondering what was the matter with the lady who was crying. Finally Scott Garrelts saw her. He didn't know what had happened either, but he went to find me.

I was lying in the training room, wishing I could join the celebration. I told Mark Letendre, "Give me some pain pills, Mark. I want to get out there."

I tried to get up, but when I stood up I thought I might pass out.

Mark said, "You look awful. Just lie down and stay still, will you?"

They wrapped my arm in ice, and I lay quietly, listening to the jubilant sounds coming from the clubhouse. Occasionally one of my teammates would come busting into the training room, and then see me lying on the table.

"Dave, what's the matter?" he would ask. "Are you hurt?"

"I'm okay. It's no big deal," I'd say. "Hey, congratulations!" I wanted to ignore my arm.

After about fifteen minutes the pain pills began to work, and my coloring came back. Dr. Campbell had examined my arm, and he said it would be all right to join the others in a little subdued celebrating. He thought I had probably dislocated the shoulder. Ever since my operation, the doctors had been concerned that without a deltoid muscle to hold the shoulder in, the joint might pop apart.

I went outside to the parking lot, where I found Janice. She said I looked like a ghost. "Everything is okay," I said. Then I went back inside to be with my teammates, champions of the National League.

A few minutes later Dr. Campbell went out to find Janice. "You poor thing," he said softly, and opened his arms wide to hug her.

The next morning I drove to Dr. Campbell's office in Palo Alto. X-rays showed I had broken my arm. By looking at film taken after the first break in Montreal, they were able to see that the new break had occurred on a hairline fracture above the main

Montreal break. Dr. Campbell thought I had probably also subluxed when I got hit—that is, my shoulder had partially and temporarily separated. He said I must have received a tremendous blow.

My prognosis was not much worse than before. My arm hadn't suffered any permanent damage; the bone would grow back stronger than ever. I had merely set my schedule back another six weeks.

But the break set back my mental state, severely.

My arm hurt more after this break than it had after Montreal, probably because I'd subluxed the shoulder. I couldn't sleep. I couldn't bathe myself. I couldn't get a coat on. I couldn't cut my meat. Janice had to do everything for me, and when she forgot, I would stand there like a hurt puppy until she noticed. I hate to ask for help.

With the World Series coming, we had friends and family visiting, people calling for tickets, reporters checking my status. Our apartment was a zoo, and I was in no shape to handle it. Janice did her best, but she was dealing with an extremely difficult person. The frustrations I couldn't tell anyone else, I vented to her. She cried. I grumbled and glared.

The World Series began five days later, in Oakland. We weren't in awe of the Athletics, but we had played them eleven times in spring training, and lost ten. That had been spring, of course, when nothing counts, but still we remembered.

We'd been underdogs all year. During spring training nobody had picked us to get into the

World Series. Nobody. So we didn't necessarily mind being in that position against the A's.

We lost two games in Oakland that weren't even close, however—the scores were 5–0 and 5–1—and we came back to Candlestick Park knowing we had a very big mountain to climb.

Maybe, we hoped, being in our own park would make the difference. I'd always hated coming to San Francisco as a San Diego Padre, because of the fans. They are loyal to the bone. Maybe their energy would jump-start us, and break a crack in the A's awesome confidence.

The weather had continued unnaturally warm. In fact, it had grown warmer, without a hint of a breeze. Ordinarily you wear a coat to Candlestick, and still freeze. But now in mid-October, it was T-shirt weather.

Feeling as I had been, it was a relief to get to the ballpark, away from the pressure cooker of our house. Janice and I were counting the days until the World Series was over. We were thrilled to be there, even feeling the way we did, but we also couldn't wait to escape the Bay Area and get home to Ohio. We badly needed to get away.

I was sitting in front of my locker, talking to Bob Knepper. He had just been out on the field snapping pictures. We felt a low rumble in the floor, sounding something like an airplane passing overhead. In the Giants' clubhouse, however, buried in concrete far beneath the stands, you can't hear airplanes. We stopped talking and looked at each other.

"That feels like an earthquake," Bob said.

"It is an earthquake," I said.

The rumbling continued and grew. The room was shaking. Players started running out the door of the clubhouse, toward the parking lot. In seconds Bob and I joined them.

By the time we had reached the open, fenced-off area just outside the stadium, the shaking had stopped. People all around were talking loudly, laughing and shaking their heads with a slightly trembly, "Wow, can you believe that?" expression on their faces. To be truthful, I hadn't felt it as dramatically as some other people did. I'd been in an earthquake in L.A. years ago that really shook me, but this hadn't seemed nearly as strong.

But then, after some time, reporters came asking for reactions. They said that the Bay Bridge was down, that a wall had collapsed in San Francisco. I began to realize that something serious had occurred. I decided that I needed to see how Janice was doing.

All the lights were out in the clubhouse and the tunnel that leads onto the field. I felt my way along in the dark, running my hands along the concrete walls and hoping not to stumble over anything, until I came out into the bright sun and green grass of the stadium.

Players and coaches from both teams were standing around talking. The stands were still half full, though oddly quiet without any music blasting from the public address system. The scoreboard was blank, dead for lack of electricity.

I peered up into the section where I knew Janice had been sitting. I located her. She was too far away to talk to me, and the aisles were jammed with people so she couldn't get near. We talked through hand signals. She made a motion of telephoning. She wanted me to phone home and see whether the kids were all right.

So I went off to find a telephone. Since the clubhouse was dark, I wouldn't be able to use a telephone there. I thought of Atlee's car phone, and I headed through the dark tunnel again, out into the parking lot looking for him. Everything was confusion. When I eventually found him, he had just come from his car. He told me it was no use. All the lines were tied up.

Going back into the stadium, I located Janice in the stands. I gestured to her: "Go home." By then it was obvious we were not going to play.

She gestured back. "No. You come with me."

Security personnel were beginning to go up into the stands, bringing wives and family members down onto the field. I asked for their assistance, and Janice, my parents, and some close friends came down.

"David, I'm really worried about Tiffany and Jonathan," Janice said. There was some panic in her voice. "I heard some people say the center of the quake was south of here. We need to get home." Foster City, south of San Francisco, was built on marshy land abutting the Bay—just the kind of land it had long been predicted would be most affected by an earthquake.

I was still in my uniform. I told them to go ahead without me, and escorted them through the long, dark tunnel to the parking lot.

* * *

I've spent so much time in that clubhouse I could find my way around in it without eyes. That is essentially what I did. There were a couple of guys with flashlights, and at critical moments in the changing process, I would ask them to shine their lights my way. Fortunately, I had worn workout clothes—no buttons to manage with my right hand. I hustled my clothes on and got back outside before Janice had even reached the car.

We began a long, quiet, anxious trip home. The traffic was completely blocked; what normally takes half an hour took two. The sun set slowly behind the mountains sweeping up from the Bay. As the light dissipated we became aware of darkness on all sides. The Bayshore freeway is normally spangled with lights along its frontage roads, while gentler lights glow from homes on the hills toward the western mountains. Now everything was blackness. The only light came from cars stacked bumper to bumper with ours, or negotiating the dark streets away from the freeway.

As we inched our way south, Janice grew more and more anxious about the children. She prayed that they would somehow have light.

We finally reached the Foster City exit. As we came over the bridge leading into our section of town, we saw the warm glow of lights. Our neighborhood was one of the very few around the Bay that had electricity.

Tiffany and Jonathan were fine. They'd been swimming when the earthquake hit. A wave of water, pushed by the earth's motion, had sloshed up and out of the pool. They had thought it was funny at first, but when the water kept sloshing back and forth, so much that they couldn't get out of the pool, they had panicked a little. One of our neighbors had gone into the pool and helped them out.

We had a full house that night. Friends and relations staying in nearby hotels had no power, and we invited them over. We didn't have much food in the house, but Janice managed to scrape together some pasta, and we had a wonderful meal. Listening to the news of our neighbors all around the Bay, we felt thankful for our lives.

Nevertheless, Janice and I went to bed that night wondering what more could happen to us.

The Tumor Is Back

A week after the earthquake, Janice, Tiffany, Jonathan, and I left San Francisco. With the emotional backwash of the earthquake, and the day-to-day delays of the World Series, the Bay Area wasn't a restful place to be. My arm was still killing me, and I hadn't been getting any sleep. I had reached such a low point emotionally that I didn't even care about the final games. I just wanted to go home to Ohio. I wanted to escape. Dr. Campbell gave us doctors' orders: Go home and get some rest.

Before we left we had to pack all our belongings and ship them home, as well as to clean our apartment. We finally got the last box to UPS. We left the place the way we'd found it: bare white walls, echoing, empty rooms.

Just before we departed, the doorbell rang. It was a deliveryman with a gift from Alex Vlahos. I hadn't seen Alex since the August 10 game, but I knew he'd gone to Seattle to have his bone marrow transplant. I'd talked to his parents and heard that the treatment had succeeded: He was clean of cancer.

Alex's gift was a huge, beautiful orchid plant,

with a note attached. "Thank you," he wrote, "for the gift of life."

We arrived in Ohio in time to catch the last of the fall colors. From our family room I could look out over our backyard into a thick stand of trees, their leaves orange and brown and red. At last the kids had a big yard and a full basement to play in, and I could actually sit quietly in a room by myself.

Two days after we got home, I had to drive up to the Cleveland Clinic for a routine MRI on my arm. I went up alone, and after doing my time in the MRI cylinder—I've become so accustomed to it that I usually sleep in there—I met with the radiologist. He showed me a big sheet of film, displaying a long series of slides. Each picture was a cross-section of my arm at a different point. As the slides traveled up my arm you could see the first break, nearly healed, and the second break, just beginning to fill in. He also pointed out a mass that had grown to fill in the area where my tumor had been removed.

I'd been aware of this mass since last July, when Dr. Muschler had last examined me. I could feel it: a lumpy, flat, firm clot of tissue.

The radiologist said he couldn't tell anything about it just by looking at the film. They'd have to analyze it, comparing it with what they'd seen before.

Janice came with me the next day. In a small examining room we met Dr. Bergfeld and Dr. Marks, an oncologist who was standing in for Dr. Muschler while he was out of town. The two of them gently removed my brace and its padding. It had been on for three weeks and was really rank. I was very glad to get it off.

Dr. Bergfeld wasn't exuberant. He wasn't booming out optimistic statements. He wasn't, in fact, talking about baseball at all. He spoke very soberly and slowly, sometimes looking down at the ground.

Both breaks, he said, seemed to be healing well. He mentioned a pitcher who had broken his arm twice, yet come back to play again. But then Dr. Bergfeld stopped and put his head down. "The problem is, David, you haven't got a muscle there. There's no muscle to support the bone."

He lifted his head, glanced at me, and went on. "But I'm not even concerned about that right now. I'm concerned about the lump. We really need to talk about these MRI results."

That was when the conversation really grew serious. Both he and Dr. Marks thought that the desmoid tumor had come back. They had no way to be sure, short of taking a biopsy, but they said that the lump was sharply defined, unlike scar tissue which tends to spread and fill in. It looked exactly like a desmoid tumor.

"Did you understand what they were saying?" Janice asked when we were in the car together, driving home. "David, do you realize that they didn't mention your future in baseball, even once?"

I didn't respond right away, because I didn't want to think about it. Throughout my life, I'd set my face toward playing baseball, pushing on no matter what the odds might be against me. That was the only way I knew to think.

"Yeah," I said finally. "It's real sobering."

"David." Janice's voice told me that she was feeling very emotional. "David, what are you going to do?"

I didn't answer her.

"David, there's so much risk. If you keep coming back, you don't know whether your arm will break again. It sounded to me as though it was more than the frozen bone. What did Dr. Bergfeld say? You don't have any muscle to support the bone. David, it could happen again. Plus the stress. It could activate the cancer. Is it worth it, David? Is it?"

"There you go again," I said, trying to joke. "Writing me off."

"David, what would you say to me if I were in your shoes? If I had cancer and I wanted to keep on with my career no matter what the risk, what would you say?"

That was easy. "I'd tell you to quit. Immediately. But Janice, you can't tell me what to do. I have to make this decision for myself."

Janice really got mad with me, as mad as I have ever seen her. She said it made her sick to her stomach to think of me going out there and taking those risks. "Enough is enough," she said. "After what we've been through in the last year, why would you do it? David, what are your motives? I know you love the game, but surely there is a point where you have to put other things ahead of baseball.

"Would you risk your arm to throw that ball again? David, does it mean that much to you?

Would you put your children through another year like this one? It's been hard on Tiffany and Jonathan. If you don't need to put them through it, why would you? What would be your motives for that? Is baseball that important to you?"

I didn't answer. I didn't say anything because I really didn't know. I knew that I wanted to keep playing. It was an instinct. No matter what, you keep on. That had been my motto. Be a tiger. Never give up. I'd had that tacked up in my locker, where I could look at it each day: "Never give up."

For the first time in our marriage, Janice wondered whether she was really ahead of baseball in my love. Ever since the broken arm in Montreal, she'd thought retirement from baseball made sense—but now, with the news that the tumor was back, she was astonished at my unwillingness to agree. I'd always said that she mattered more to me than baseball, that she was number one in my life. But had that been easy to say so long as I didn't have to choose? When push came to shove, would I put baseball ahead of her? Ahead of our kids? Ahead of my life?

I just didn't know. I called up Atlee the next day. I told Atlee what the doctors had said. We'd talked about retirement many times, starting way back when I was disabled with a sore shoulder. Atlee had always wanted me to stay in the game. I'm not sure whether he wanted that for sound, objective reasons, or just because he didn't want to play without me around. Maybe it was both. At any rate, I expected him to tell me to keep on—or at least to wait until spring training, and see how my arm felt then.

He was somber when he heard about the tumor, however. I described Janice's question—"What would you say if I were in your shoes?" He thought that was a very interesting angle. "I never thought of it," he said. "But if Jenny had a tumor, I know exactly what I'd say. I'd tell her to quit."

How do you quit, though? How do you leave something you love, something that has been your life? Perhaps you quit one thing only when something else begins to make a stronger appeal.

As I thought about the possibility of retiring, as I let that idea take root in my mind, I was surprised to find that it brought me peace rather than turmoil. That threw me a little.

I began imagining life without baseball. I would miss the game, but I could take up other sports. I love to play golf. I didn't think I'd mind clobbering that tiny white ball.

And the thought of not getting on an airplane again, not leaving my family, the thought of settling down in Youngstown and living quietly—that was profoundly attractive.

Janice's question about my motives made me think. Why would I continue? What would I gain, driving myself and my family through another comeback? What did I have to gain in baseball that I hadn't already gained? It wasn't the money. I wasn't interested in attention, and even if I were, I doubted that I could ever achieve any more attention than I'd had during the past year.

COMEBACK

It came down to this: I would miss the game. And I would miss my friends.

A week after coming home to Youngstown, Janice and I had to leave again. Long before, we had committed ourselves to several California speaking engagements, to be done as soon as the season was over. One was a prayer breakfast in Santa Cruz, the city most decimated by the earthquake. We hated to leave home again. I really didn't feel that I'd been able to rest, with the phone calls, the doctor visits, and the medical issues to sort through. But we didn't believe that we could cancel. So we got on the plane.

Surprisingly, the trip provided just the shot of renewal we needed. We saw wonderful old friends, and were able to talk to large audiences about our lives and our faith. Taking the focus off our own problems, we tried to reach out to others. That lifted our spirits.

While I was in San Diego I talked with a long-time close friend about the possibility of retirement. The more I talked, the more retirement appealed to me. The conviction gradually came. I needed to do it. I wanted to do it.

I don't think Janice completely believed me until I told Atlee, though. From San Diego Janice and I went up to the Bay Area, speaking in a church, traveling to Santa Cruz for a prayer breakfast, and speaking at a wild, fun rock concert. On Friday Atlee drove me up to Candlestick Park. I was going to have some pictures taken for the cover of this book. On the way I told him that I had made the decision.

He was thoughtful in response—shocked a bit, I think. "It's interesting," he said. "Bob Knepper called me yesterday, and we talked specifically about you. Bob told me he was praying that you would have peace about retiring from baseball."

For a moment Atlee said nothing. "I couldn't pray that way for you," he said. "I didn't know what you ought to do. I've just been praying that you would experience peace in whatever God led you to decide. I want you to be at peace, Dave."

"I am, Atlee," I said. "It's as though a tremendous pressure has been released."

When we got back to his house, Atlee asked Janice if she was happy about the decision. I could see her struggle with her answer. She was happy, yes—happy that I would be home, happy that we could concentrate on the tumor without trying to think about a future in baseball as well. But for all four of us, the full meaning of retirement began to hit. There would be no more baseball together.

We had a soft, sad, radiant evening with Atlee and Jenny. It was tremendously fun, tremendously satisfying to our souls. Yet we were grieving, too. We were saying good-bye—good-bye to the life we'd lived together in baseball. We'd spent so many hours together. We'd been so close. Atlee had been the guy with whom I'd gone through the batting order each game, discussing how to pitch to every last guy in the National League. Atlee had been the guy who would call me fifteen minutes after he'd dropped me off home from a night game—calling me because he had thought of one last thing he had to say.

That night, after we'd prayed together and said

good-bye, after Janice and I had climbed into our hotel bed and pulled the covers up, I lay in the darkness thinking.

"What am I going to do about Atlee?" I said to Janice. "My buddy Atlee, what am I going to do?"

Was It Worth It?

A few days after we got back to Youngstown, we went out to dinner in Pittsburgh and arrived home just in time to catch the ending of *The Natural,* a baseball movie starring Robert Redford. The baby-sitter had it on, and I was instantly hooked.

What caught my eye was the stadium. The movie was filmed in Buffalo, New York, where I'd played for two years in Double-A baseball. It's a grand, old, classically-styled stadium, with tall, brooding stands. It brought back memories.

"Remember that infield?" I asked Janice, as we watched Robert Redford come to bat. "Boy, that was brutal. We called it the Rockyard, didn't we?"

"Where's the wall?" she asked. "Remember the right field wall?"

"Two hundred and eighty-five feet, down the line," I said. "A pitcher's nightmare. Remember, we had a guy who led the league in home runs one year, because he was a left-handed pull hitter and hit to that wall all the time."

We watched the movie closely, and saw that they had repainted the number on the wall, making the distance 310 feet instead of 285.

"Remember the rats?" she asked.

"Oh, the rats." The ballpark was in a terrible neighborhood, where you feared for your life walking on the streets. "Boy, that was a happy time. Wasn't it?"

We watched to the ending. The Robert Redford character, an old ballplayer who has come back for one last game, hits a towering home run high up over the outfield wall, striking the light pole and shattering the bulbs so they rain down in sparks like fireworks. The ball keeps traveling, on into the night, until it lands magically in a baseball mitt—and we see that it has been caught by Robert Redford's son, who is playing catch with him.

I thought, "That's me. That's my career."

I'd had a chance to hit one last home run, so to speak. Now I would be playing catch with my kids, just as my dad had done with me. Baseball ends where it began: with a father and a son, throwing the ball around.

Two days later I made my retirement official. I called Al Rosen and told him to place me on the roster of retired players. Al said he was grieving over my decision. He said he would miss me. Within a few hours I was facing a battery of TV cameras in my living room, telling the world what I'd decided and why.

There were many reasons, of course, not the least of which was my desire to be with my family, and not to put them through another grueling attempt at playing ball. I also felt it was time to move on—to get started on the new life I believe God has planned for me. I've always enjoyed giving financially to causes I believe in, and I am really looking forward to giving my *self* as well. How I'll do that, what my precise job will be, I don't know. I like the idea of coaching at a college level, with the chance to have an impact on the lives of young men.

The key factor was the recurrence of the tumor. I will have surgery again, and there is no certainty at all that a second operation will eliminate the problem. Desmoid tumors can come back after second surgeries, third surgeries, any number of surgeries. My doctors have continued to emphasize that my life is not at risk, but they've been frank to tell me that I may be in treatment for a long time. The ultimate decision, if nothing else succeeds, would be to amputate my arm. We're far, far away from that as of yet, but if it comes to it, I'll be ready.

Considering all that, another comeback had become so improbable as to seem impossible. I'm a realist. I don't need to play baseball. Other things, such as my family, are far more important.

Will I miss baseball? I suspect that when spring comes, and I talk on the telephone to Atlee about how he's pitching, and the weather in Ohio is warming up, I'll wish I could be there. I'll see somebody pitch and think, *It could be me.*

I really don't believe, though, that I'll struggle with it. I've always thought that my life was a lot more than baseball. It is just a game, after all—a great one, but still a game.

I won't miss the attention and glamor one bit. Memory is short, and it won't be long before, outside of Youngstown at least, my baseball feats won't be remembered. That isn't going to bother me. I will be very happy watching my family grow in this little town, doing whatever work God has called me to do.

There's a bittersweet quality to my retirement, of course—as perhaps there is to all retirements. Inevitably, "what-if" kinds of questions come up. What if I had recognized the symptoms of a hairline fracture in Montreal, and quit before my arm broke? Perhaps I would have pitched in the World Series then. Perhaps I could have made a difference.

Or "what if" I had never contracted cancer in my throwing arm? What kind of success might have come to me?

I don't think about such questions, though. To me my comeback had perfect timing. I could have broken my arm in Stockton. Or I could have lost my three minor league games, and stayed down there indefinitely.

The way I see it, my comeback was written better than a movie script. In fact, if it were a movie script, it would probably be discarded as unbelievable.

Was the comeback worth it? Some people have asked whether it was worth struggling for that whole year, in order to pitch only twice at the major league level. Was it worth it, considering how it ended in pain?

I don't even have to hesitate. Yes, it was worth it, a million times over. It was an unparalleled thrill. When I think of my years in baseball I put those games in Stockton, San Francisco, and Montreal at the very top.

Was It Worth It?

I got to live out the greatest boyhood dream of all. I got to do what the experts said was impossible, to come back from cancer and pitch a major league baseball game. Without a deltoid muscle in my pitching arm, I won a game in a pennant drive in front of tens of thousands of screaming fans. What more would anybody want out of baseball? The fans who supported me—who screamed for me, prayed for me, wrote to me—they knew that it was worth it.

It was worth it on another level too. It was worth it because of the growth it brought in my life.

I've learned a lot in the past two years. I've learned how precious my wife and my children are. They were always important, but never so precious to me as they are now.

I've learned how important it is to serve other people. Time and again, I have been astonished and humbled by the loving concern people have shown me. I don't think I'll be the same after experiencing that.

Perhaps most of all, I've learned to put my life in God's hands. The hardest part of the last two years has been the uncertainty. I had to learn to do what was within my grasp, one day at a time, and leave control of the rest trustingly to God.

Such are the lessons that come when a man faces adversity. I don't think I could have gained them in any other way.

I'm clearly not done with adversity. My future is as unknown as before. All I can say for certain is that I'm done playing baseball.

There are times in the baseball season, during the dog days of summer, when the six months of the schedule seem like six years. You don't want to play baseball. Your body is tired and your spirit is weary, but you have to keep on. You go out and do your best. That's called maturity. That's what is required of me as I face my next operation, and whatever may come afterwards.

I leave baseball with a great sense of satisfaction. When I think back on my career, I do so with a big, fat smile on my face. How could I feel anything else?

Every year in America hundreds of thousands of kids go out to play Little League, and every year each of them dreams of playing in the major leagues. The odds are so slim. It's as if you had a huge stadium jammed full of kids, each wearing a uniform and a glove, and just one out of all those thousands got picked to come down onto the field and play with the big boys.

I was that kid. I got to play with the big boys. And even more: I got the chance to come back.

Postscript

ON January 4, 1990, I underwent surgery at Memorial Sloan Kettering Hospital in New York. Dr. Murray Brennan, chief of surgery there, cut open my left arm and removed the tumor that had grown where the first one had been removed. All my remaining deltoid muscle was taken out, along with a portion of my triceps muscle. If Jaws had taken a good-sized nibble in the first surgery, this time my upper left arm looks as though he got a full bite.

Though the tumor was next to my humerus bone, very near to the fracture, it did not seem to have invaded the bone. Only time will tell for certain. During at least the next two years, I will be reexamined every three months. Given the nature of desmoid tumors, no one can rule out the possibility of a recurrence.

To reduce the possibility of cancer coming back, my doctors used brachytherapy. This is a kind of radiation treatment that Sloan Kettering has pioneered. During my surgery, thin catheter tubes were sewn inside my arm. A few days later, pellets of radioactive iridium were inserted into these tubes. For five days I was isolated from doctors, nurses, relatives, and friends, to prevent them from being exposed to the radiation. Brachytherapy provided strong doses of radiation directly from within my wound, where cancer cells were most likely to remain. When the five days were up, the tubes were removed.

I really didn't like being isolated for five days, but it provided time to meditate and pray. I thought a great deal about the life of people who are in prison, isolated far longer than I was. I also thought about patients and their families whom I was meeting at Sloan Kettering. Most of them were facing sickness and adversity that made my case seem almost trivial. They helped me remember how little reason I had to feel sorry for myself. They also helped me realize again how fragile and precious life is. I remembered the same truth Bob Knepper brought home to me in Montreal: the greatest miracle of all is the miracle of life in Jesus Christ.

There is no guarantee that I will get well, that I will overcome cancer, even that I will live another ten minutes. But Jesus Christ, the son of God, was crucified and three days later rose from the dead, conquering death forevermore. As the Bible teaches in John 3:16, anyone who believes in Jesus will not perish, but have everlasting life. He is the ground of my peace. With him, I can face any adversity.

Therefore we do not lose heart. Though outwardly we are wasting away, yet inwardly we are being renewed day by day. For our light and momentary troubles are achieving for us an eternal glory that far outweighs them all.

Postscript

So we fix our eyes not on what is seen, but on what is unseen. For what is seen is temporary, but what is unseen is eternal.

—2 Corinthians 4:16–18

The publishers gratefully acknowledge the contributions of the following photographers and other sources: the San Francisco Giants Organization; the San Diego Padres Organization; Dennis Desprois; Wide World Photos, Inc.; Mickey Pfleger; *Sports Illustrated*, Time Inc.; Kim Komenich, Craig Lee, *The San Francisco Examiner*; John Taylor, Journal de Montréal; Fred Vuich; LIFE-SAVERS FOUNDATION OF AMERICA; Pat Johnson; KNBR Radio 68, San Francisco, the flagship station of San Francisco Giants baseball; Stephen Dunn; Focus West; Seattle FilmWorks. All Scripture quotations taken from the *Holy Bible: New International Version* (North American Edition) are copyrighted © 1973, 1978, 1984, by The International Bible Society. Used by permission of Zondervan Bible Publishers.